# The Educator's Guide to Teaching Methodologies

***Marilyne Gustafson***

*Editors:*

*Donna Wright*
*Christine Ramos*

Creative Healthcare Management, Minneapolis, MN

For permission requests or ordering information, write to the publisher at:
Creative Healthcare Management
1701 East 79th Street, Suite 1
Minneapolis, MN 55425-1151
or call 1-800-728-7766 or (952) 854-9015. [fax: 952-854-1866]

Creative Healthcare Management can also be contact through e-mail and the Internet.
E-mail address: chcm@chcm.com
Internet location: http://www.chcm.com

Printed in the United States of America.

Publisher's Cataloging-in-Publication Data:

Gustafson, Marilyne

Educator's Guide to Teaching Methodologies

ISBN: 0-9621520-9-9

Cover photos depict the following methodologies:

Upper left photo: Self Defense education poster
Upper right photo: "The Princess and the Chemo Spill" fairy tale
Lower left photo: Dysrhythmias self learning packet
Lower right photo: Hematology Jeopardy game

Cover design and graphic artist: Jeanne Kosfeld
Photographer: Nancy Mellgren
Copy editing: Tracey Maassen, Chris Bjork
Model in photos: Donna Wright

# About the Author

Marilyne Gustafson, RN, Ph.D., has over 38 years experience in education. She has served as faculty at the University of Minnesota, the University of Michigan, and at Mounds Midway Diploma Nursing Program. She received her Bachelors of Science in Nursing Education from the University of Minnesota, a Masters of Science from the University of Colorado, and her Ph.D. from Walden University in Naples, FL.

Marilyne has published and lectured on a variety of topics related to continuing education and the use of creative methods in education. She has authored many articles including a series in the Journal of Continuing Education in Nursing. Her work has been used in a variety of settings, both in health care and non-health care settings. She has a wonderful gift for seeing application of both traditional and nontraditional methodologies, and including multicultural aspects in her work.

Marilyne Gustafson has dedicated her professional life to providing quality, creative education. She has done this through her own creative teaching approaches, as well as her dedication to mentoring others. Her work has had a profound impact on her students, who are now teachers in many corners of the world.

# Preface

The development of guidelines for nurse educators evolved over a number of years when Sheila Corcoran-Perry and I were teaching graduate students in courses dealing with the teaching/learning process. The guidelines were intended to be just that -- a guide for those seeking basic information about methodologies and/or new ways to approach or combine approaches to a well known and well used strategy. The outline format was selected because it provides a quick reference which would require minimal reading and it would also provide an easy way to identify key concepts quickly.

I found that the guidelines could combine ideas from education and nursing, providing the nurse educator with examples when appropriate and available. Some very "old, tried and true" methods were placed alongside those which might be "new and untried."

The guidelines are not intended to be all inclusive. I tried to include research findings whenever they were available. The need for research about teaching strategies is apparent as some of the strategies not only have limited sources, but they also have limited or no research to support their use.

The term nurse educator is used broadly to include a variety of nurses and other health care educators who teach in a variety of settings, levels, and programs.

Creative teaching methods are needed in nursing and healthier education. The possibilities for additional guidelines are limitless. Until then, I trust these will be helpful, and that you will be encouraged to try many of them.

Marilyne Backlund Gustafson

# Table of Contents

# ALLEGORY

## Definition

Allegory is a fictitious narrative used as a vehicle of truth, although not always moral or religious truth.

## Purposes

- An intended or sustained metaphor in which concrete objects are made to represent things spiritual in order to present high truths with vividness and power.
- To entertain, instruct, one form of satire.

---

**Advantages**

- Those familiar with the form (English, Hindu) may identify it as a valuable story telling form.
- Similar to a parable in advantages
- A potentially useful form of oral traditional sharing

**Disadvantages**

- Much less known today.
- May be difficult to obtain examples.
- Need to know the primitive people's standards for development and conduct.

---

## Points to Remember

- Doesn't need interpretation -- it is a stand alone teaching tool.
- The narrative and its interpretation are interwoven.

**Other Related Methodologies:** Parable

## References

Nowlin, C. The story teller and his pack (pp. 246-266). Springfield, MA: Milton Bradley Co., 1929. (An old, but quite complete source about this method.)

(Example: Hans Christian Anderson's, Ugly Duckling).

# ANALOGY

**Definition**

*Analogy* is a resemblance in some particulars between things otherwise unlike; a resemblance of principle between objects, situations or ideas superficially unlike.

**Purposes**

- Explain unknown concepts by comparing them to similar but more familiar concepts.
- Make the abstract more concrete.
- Provide structure for new information.
- Develop conceptual abilities.
- Generate creativity.

---

**Advantages**

- A powerful teaching tool to stimulate insight and creativity.
- Can be used to make the unfamiliar familiar or the familiar unfamiliar.
- Supplement verbal instruction.
- Spark active learning.
- Useful for a wide variety of teaching situations and disciplines.
- Provides for culturally relevant examples.
- Teacher can gauge learner's understanding.
- May be used in problem solving situations.

**Disadvantages**

- Appropriateness is based on knowledge of learner's background, experience, and culture.
- Young children may have difficulty with something being like rather than the thing itself.
- Difficult, generally, for the mentally retarded to grasp.

---

**Points to Remember**

- Need to be familiar with the concept to be taught.
- The more informed about the learners, the easier it is to come up with comparable events, processes, objects.
- Knowledge of the learner is imperative (consider age, educational level, ethnic origin, experiences, occupation, etc.).
- Use learners' daily experiences for ideas.
- May ask learners to think of their own analogies.
- Right side of brain promotes analogous, contextual thinking.

**Other Related Methodologies:** Metaphor

## References

Alexander, P., White, C., Haensley, P., & Crimnins-Jeanes, M. (1987). Training in analogical reasoning. American Educational Research Journal, 24 (3). 387-404.

Deshler, D. (1985). Metaphor and values in higher education. Academe, 71 (6).

Fuszard, B. (1989). Innovative teaching strategies in nursing. Rockville, MD: Aspen. pp. 281-288.

Elsberry, N., & Sorensen, M. (1986). Using analogies in patient teaching. Am. Journal Of Nursing, 86 (10). 1171-1172.

Jorgensen, S. (1980). Using analogies to develop conceptual abilities. Paper presented at the Annual Meeting of the Association for Educational Communications and Technology, Denver, CO, April, 1980.

Joyce, B., & Weil, M. (1972). Synectics: a model to develop creativity in models of teaching. Englewood Cliffs, NJ: Prentice Hall.

Werner, D., & Bower, B. (1982). Helping health workers learn. Palo Alto, CA: Hesperian Foundation.

Joyce & Weil. (1986). Steps of synectic model of teaching using analogy. (pp. 182-183).

Summary of Steps:

Phase One: Description of Present Condition
Teacher has student describe situation or topic as they see it now.

Phase Two: Direct Analogy
Student suggestions direct analogies, select one, and explore (describe) it further.

Phase Three: Personal Analogy
Students "become" the analogy they selected in phase two.

Phase Four: Compressed Conflict
Students take their descriptions from phases two and three, suggest several compressed conflicts, and choose one.

Phase Five: Direct Analogy
Students generate and select another direct analogy based on the compressed conflict.

Phase Six: Re-examination of the Original Task
Teacher has students move back to original task or problem and use the last analogy and/or the entire synectics experience.

# AUDIO MAP

**Definition**

*Audio map* is a cassette used to give information on a self-guided tour. (Combines audio cassette and map.)

**Purposes**

- Provide an auditory explanation of what is being seen.
- Serve as a guide to learners.

---

**Advantages**

- Provides verbal description of details.
- Allows for self-pacing on tour.
- Releases tour guide/teacher.
- Inexpensive.
- May be used with either a walking or driving tour.
- Avoids boredom of repeated description by guide.

**Disadvantages**

- Preparation is time consuming.
- May be frustrating if equipment is difficult to operate or nonfunctioning.
- Must be periodically updated.
- If equipment is damaged, may be expensive.

---

**Points to Remember**

- Content to be placed on audiomap needs to be carefully planned.
- Length, sound effects, and interest must be considered.
- Teacher or preparer must try out initially and periodically.
- Instructions on how to operate the equipment must be clear and as simple as possible.
- May wish to have an opportunity to discuss, comment, and/or evaluate.

**Other Related Methodologies:** Audio Tape, Map, Self-Tour Guidelines

**References**

Audiomaps on cassette give personal guided tours. (1980, January). UPI, Miami Herald. (Describes guided tours of Scottish landscape features.)

## Definition

*Audio tape* is a recorded sound on magnetic tape (cassette).
Since "audio" can refer to a wide range of equipment, from homemade audiocassette to satellite, and since cassette players are used much more widely than reel-to-reel players, the cassette player has been selected for discussion here.

## Purposes

- Enables learners to overcome obstacles of time and space so that they can relive original experience when they choose.
- Communicates a message -- lecture, report, music, other sounds.
- Self-improvement -- teaches communication skills and enhances verbal presentations.

## Disadvantages

- Communication of a recorded event is delayed.
- Learners may need to be helped to grasp meaning from auditory stimuli; it is a complex skill.
- Poorly prepared or poorly used materials may distract or discourage learners.
- The existence of many kinds of recorders may mean that an individual who thinks he/she knows how to operate the equipment may do so incorrectly, resulting in delay or possible erasing
- Equipment must function well. If an electrical outlet is not handy, charged batteries will be needed.
- Time must be taken to preview and select appropriate commercial tapes.
- Time is required to write and rewrite scripts.

---

## Advantages

- Tape allows flexible timing and spacing of instruction.
- It is inexpensive, simple, and reusable.
- Its convenience is threefold-easy to handle, store and transport.
- Tapes can be purchased ready-made, or can be homemade.
- Versatile use may include travel, field trips, spontaneous occasions.
- Tape is equally useful in small or large groups.
- Children and the handicapped can operate cassette players.
- Tape can be integrated with visual media.
- Use can extend beyond the classroom to at-home study.
- Tape recording encourages creativity of learners and teacher.
- "Professional" voices can be substituted for a teacher's in tape preparation.
- Tape is under the teacher's control--he/she may stop, replay, interlace.

## Suggestions for Preparation

- Plan carefully in producing tapes.
- Presentations must deal with the subject and be well organized.
- The teacher must know how to operate each piece of equipment.
- Read the instructions first; then:
  a. Pay attention to acoustics. Acoustical quality depends on absorption and reverberation.
  b. Prepare tape in a room with carpeting and draperies rather than tile floors and hard walls, if you have a choice.
  c. Make the message as interesting as possible.
  d. Stop mind drifting by:
     (1) Changing rhythm or texture every 30-60 seconds (change of voice, shift in emphasis, sound effect, or musical break).
     (2) Using 5-6 minutes maximum for sub topics.
  e. If you're using a long tape or several in a series, accompany it with a printed text. It may include index, approximate lengths or locations of various passages, brief review between sections or at the end to reinforce or summarize.
  f. Practice.

**Points to Remember**

- Plan carefully how you will use the tape.
- Proper use depends on good listening skills, and you may need to teach discriminative listening.
- Remember that motivation is essential to attentive listening.
- Effectiveness depends on how well the material is introduced and discussed.
- Practice using the equipment before class. Don't assume it is just like a similar machine.
- There are audiovisual books that provide detailed instruction on operations, cleaning, purchase, repair, and storage of cassettes (filing cabinets for cassettes may be necessary for large supplies).

**Other Related Methodologies:** Listening Centers; Audio Tutorial; Self-pacing Learning Centers.

**References**

Cooper, S. (1980). Methods of teaching revisited, audio tape recordings. Journal of Continuing Education in Nursing, 11 (6), 20-27.

Evans, A. D., et al. (1980, May). Speech compression: Options for speeding nursing education. Journal of Nursing Education, 19 (5), 20-26. (Audio tapes are compressed -- reasons are given.)

Fredette, S. L. Individualized clinical teaching via the tape recorder. Image, 26 (3), 80-83.

Kinder, J. (1973). Using instructional media. (pp. 114-134). New York: D. Van Nostrand. (Excellent resource on use of cassette recordings.)

Koch, H. B. (1975). Audio: The oldest medium. Nursing Outlook, 23 (7), 419. (Briefly discusses the audio medium and value of audio taping.)

McGrane, H. F. (1975). Tape recorded evaluation: A method of teaching. Journal of Nursing Education, 14 (1), 11-17. (Suggests one use of tape recordings in nursing education.)

Vogt, R. B. (1980, April). Enhancing students' experience through the use of tape recordings. Journal of Nursing Education, 19 (4), 51-53. (Used as a teaching tool in clinical teaching.)

Wittmeyer, A. (1971). Teaching by audio tape. Nursing Outlook, 19 (3), 162-163. (Helpful in looking at one baccalaureate program's use of audio tapes.)

## Definition

*Annotated Bibliography* is a list of books, articles, and pamphlets that contain useful information about a particular subject being studied and one in which each item is briefly described.

## Purposes

- Provide the reader with more detailed information about the content than is supplied by the title.

## Individuals who may Prepare the Annotated List

- A member in the learning group may be asked or volunteer.
- A member of a planning committee or workshop may assume responsibility.
- A speaker, panel member or other resource person involved in the program may be requested by the planning group to prepare it.
- A teacher, speaker, resource person, or other individual may identify a need for the annotated list.

## Obtaining Ready-made Lists

- Books and articles contain ready-made lists. They may be used alone, incorporated into revisions, or be the stimulus for an original list.
- Public libraries, school, college, and university libraries are logical sources: for both materials and individuals who can assist.
- National organizations may have ready-made lists, as well as publishers, industry, and other agencies.
- Some county and state organizations have ready lists, collections of materials, and pamphlets available.
- Large libraries, especially those with media resources and interagency affiliations are likely to have resources of both individuals and media resource and equipment. This source may be useful in locating international materials and otherwise difficult-to-obtain and/or infrequently requested materials.

## Suggestions for Use

- Relate selection to the objectives of the session or course.
- The list should not be so long as to be overwhelming. 10-20 carefully selected and appropriate titles are usually enough.
- Give the list an attractive title. Humor may be helpful. Try to avoid a forbidding phrase like "An Annotated Bibliography."

- Initiate interest in the subject.
- Strive for accuracy and completeness. Use complete titles of articles and books, names and dates. Do not abbreviate unless the journal is very well known (i.e., Am. Journal Of Nursing). Include all pertinent data to assist rapid location of the materials. It may be useful to include volume, number, complete date, cost, availability in paperback, address of unknown publisher (street and zip, please). If materials are available in more than one source (i.e., readings, books, digests) this may save time and expense in location.
- Consider whether there is a need for the material to be quite recent and contemporary in nature vs. historical.
- Determine if the nature of the material is such that divergent points of view should be included.
- Begin preparation far enough in advance if comprehensiveness is important. If several (more than one) individuals are contributing to the list, assign a deadline date to each contributor.

**Points to Remember**

- Prepare sufficient quality and quantity.
- Determine if the cost is assumed in the cost of the meeting or conference. If not, determine what is a reasonable cost and inform participants what that cost is going to be.
- Consider (or get suggestions) distributing the annotated list prior to the session if advance study is desired. (Then instruct them to bring them to the meeting if they will need them and prepare extra copies for those who forget to bring them along.)
- Check with the speaker(s) or resource persons if they have preferences for distribution before, during, or after the presentation.
- Explain the rationale for the list and where difficult-to-locate items may be obtained.
- It may be helpful to encourage members to use the list and to refer to it several times during the session(s). Several speakers may wish to refer to the same list, if appropriate.
- Group members may be good sources of comment or recommendation about the list. (Be prepared for some negative or unexpected ones, as well as positive recommendations.)
- Do not assume that distributing an annotated reading list will insure that members have been able to locate and/or read the references.
- Include feedback about the list in the evaluation plans.

**Other Related Methodologies:** Reading List

**References**

Bergevin, P., Morris, D., & Smith, R. M. (1963). Adult education procedures. New York: Seabury Press.

Cooper, S. (1983). Methods of teaching revisited: handouts and reading lists. Journal of Continuing Education in Nursing, 14 (2), 36-38.

# BRAINSTORMING

## Definition

*Brainstorming* is a popular non-technical term for certain techniques for the stimulation of creative thinking in the development of new ideas; consists of individual or, more generally, small group activity in which a deliberate attempt is made to think uncritically but creatively about all possible solutions to a given problem. This involves groups participating in spontaneous and unrestrained discussion. (Good)

## Purposes

- Promote creative thinking.
- Develop a quantity of ideas.
- Broaden perspectives beyond the typical or usual.

---

**Advantages**

- Distinguishes creative and critical thinking. In brainstorming creative thinking is used, withholding critical thinking until later.
- Having quantity of ideas as a goal promotes freer sharing of "silly ideas."
- Promotes "hitchhiking" on ideas.
- Provides for pooling of ideas.
- Focus on quantity of ideas increases the probability of ideas with quality being shared as well.
- Supplement to individual thinking.

**Disadvantages**

- Time consuming.
- Not appropriate for problems requiring value judgments.
- Is not complete in itself. Requires follow-up with critical thinking and decision-making.
- Requires orientation and practice.

---

## Format

- Break down a complex problem into problems specific enough to be brainstormed.
- Have each individual brainstorm ideas or solutions first for a designated length of time (2-5 minutes).
- Use Osborn's (1963) rules for brainstorming.
  a. Criticism is ruled out: Judgment is suspended until a later screening or evaluation session. Allowing yourself to be critical at the same time you are being creative is like trying to get hot and cold water from one faucet at the same time. Ideas aren't hot enough; criticism isn't cold enough -- results are tepid.

b. Free Wheeling is welcomed:
   The wilder the ideas, the better. Even offbeat, impractical suggestions may "trigger" practical suggestions which might not otherwise occur.
c. Quantity is wanted:
   The greater the number of ideas, the greater likelihood a good idea will emerge. It is easier to pare down a long list of ideas than puff up a short list.
d. Combination and Improvement are sought:
   Two or more ideas can be combined into a still better idea.

- Questions which help spur ideas include:
  a. Put to other uses? New ways to use as is? Other uses if modified?
  b. Adapt? What else is like this? What other ideas does this suggest?
  c. Modify? Change meaning, color, motion, sound, odor, taste, form, shape?
  d. Magnify? What to add? Greater frequency? Stronger? Larger? Plus ingredient?
  e. Minify? What to subtract? Eliminate? Smaller? Lighter? Slower? Split up? Less frequent?
  f. Substitute? Who else instead? What else instead? Other place or time?
  g. Rearrange? Other layout? Other sequence? Change pace?
  h. Reverse? Opposites? Turn it backward? Upside-down? Inside-out?
  i. Combine? How about a blend, an assortment? Combine purposes? Combine ideas?
- After individuals have brainstormed, then ideas can be pooled in a group brainstorming effort.

**References**


Bouchard, T. J., & Hare, M. (1970). Size, performance and potential in brainstorming groups. Journal of Applied Psychology, 54 (1), 51-55. (Group brainstorming, over range of group sizes, inhibits rather than facilitates creative thinking and pooled individual effort is far more productive than group effort.)

Collaros, P. A., & Anderson, L. R. (1969). Effects of perceived expertness upon creativity of members of brainstorming groups. Journal of Applied Psychology, 53, 159-163. (Perceived expertise of other members makes a brainstorming group less effective than the pooled results of members working alone. Study uses three groups with findings suggesting careful attention to the selection of members.)

Cooper, S. (1978). Methods of teaching-revisited, brainstorming. Journal of Continuing Education in Nursing, 9 (6), 16-18.

DeTornyay, R. (1971). Strategies for teaching nursing (pp. 97). New York: John Wiley.

Good, C. V. Dictionary of education (3rd ed.). New York: McGraw-Hill.

Osborn, A. F. (1963). Applied imagination (3rd ed.). New York: Charles Scribner & Sons.

# BULLETIN BOARD

## Definition

*Bulletin Board* is a board to which can be fastened pictures or other materials intended for display. (Good)

## Purposes

- Communicate news and information.
- Attract and hold attention.
- Affect attitudes and develop involvement about a variety of topics.
- Encourage learning and produce action.
- A tool to introduce material, reinforce desired learning and motivate.

---

**Advantages**

- Inexpensive, easy to update.
- Allows for variety in ideas presented and materials used.
- Flexible, portable.
- Uses short periods of time for learning.
- Allows for individual pacing, slow learners may spend the time needed and/or return.
- A way to provide supplementary materials.
- Allows for creativity.
- May utilize the talents of learners; both their ideas and products.
- Versatile; may be very simple or very elaborate.

**Disadvantages**

- Takes some time to design and create.

---

## Points to Remember

- Keep it simple -- neat and organized. Be concerned with layout and design.
- Make sure the goal is clear.
- Keep it up-to-date.
- Change often! Remove and return material rather than leaving it too long. (2-14 days - over 2 weeks is generally too long.)
- Use color to attract attention and curiosity.
- Use interesting designs, drawings, diagrams, pictures, photos, charts, cartoons.
- Be sure the lettering is large enough to be readable. You may create interest with a catchy headline or title.
- Use humor.
- You may wish to have a board for teaching purposes separate from a board for messages.
- Placement can be very important and a portable board may serve your purposes best.
- To be effective, it requires time, effort, and planning.

- It may be wise to have one person responsible for a period of time.
- Use variety in texture, dimension, and color.

**Basic Materials Necessary**

1. For Bulletin Boards:
   a. Cork (or cork tiles), soft wood covered with flannel, felt, or burlap.
   b. Inexpensive boards may be made from heavy cardboard or plywood covered with suitable fabric.
2. Materials and Ideas:
   a. Illustrative materials may be elaborate, expensive commercially prepared ones, or inexpensive clippings from a variety of sources (magazines -- popular and professional, newspapers, brochures, pamphlets, photographs (Polaroid), posters, graphs, cartoons, maps--) to name a few.
   b. Materials which are three-dimensional or direct objectives add interest.
   c. May want to have files (and a filing system) to collect and organize materials for ready and repeated use.

**Teacher Responsibilities**

- Plan for the effective use of the board and/or encourage learners to assume that responsibility.
- Collect and organize materials for preparing the board--illustrations, lettering materials, felt pens, paper, poster board, etc.
- Encourage creative viewing and planning if learners are to be held responsible for learning from the board.

**Other Related Methodologies:** Tackboard

**References**

Cooper, S. S. (1975). The bulletin board as a learning resource. Journal of Continuing Education in Nursing, 6 (3), 51-55. (An especially helpful article for ideas for the inservice educator.)

Dale, E. (1969). Audiovisual methods in teaching (3rd ed., pp. 330-335). New York: The Dryden Press, Holt, Rinehart & Winston.

Good, C. V. (1973). Dictionary of education (3rd ed.). New York: McGraw-Hill.

McCune, H. L., & Meyer, R. T. (1954). The bulletin board -- An effective teaching aid. Nursing Outlook, 7 (9), 532-533. (Suggests several inexpensive materials for both making the board and objects to place on the board.)

## BUZZ GROUP

**Definition**

*Buzz Group* is a method of dividing a large group into small groups of 5-10 for a limited time to work on a specific problem. (6 people working for 6 minutes leads to the term "discussion 66")

**Purposes**

- Discuss a presentation, define and/or analyze a problem.
- Prepare questions for the next general session.
- Express learning needs and evaluate learning experiences.

---

**Advantages**

- Involves all members of a group.
- Creates an atmosphere of informality.
- Usually leaves the group enthusiastic.
- Can be used on any size large group.
- Small groups save time.
- Leader can structure activities.
- Small group can refine and assign priorities for total group.
- Provides new ideas.
- Can provide feedback to teacher regarding content and process.

**Disadvantages**

- Time is limited.
- If directions aren't clear, group can waste time.
- May be difficult to achieve consensus.

---

**Points to Remember**

- Leader usually announces purpose, how to divide the total group, time allowed and what they are expected to report.
- Roles such as spokesperson and recorder may be used and should be selected by the small group.
- Written report may be requested (such as on board).
- Physical facility must be capable of accommodations of quick small group formation.
- Directions must be clear, specific, and succinct.

**References**

Knowles, M. (1959). Informal adult education. Newark, NJ: Associated Press.

O'Connor, A. (1986). Nursing staff development and continuing education Boston: Little, Brown & Co.

# CARTOONS AND COMICS

## Definition

*Cartoon* is an interpretive picture that makes use of symbolism, often with bold exaggeration, to present at a glance a message or point of view concerning events, people, or situations.
*Comic strip* is a serial or continuous comical pictorial story through a series of drawings. Also known as strip drawings.

## Purposes

- Tells a story with pictures and symbols.
- Captures interest.
- Facilitates learning.
- Increases understanding of concepts.
- Utilizes humor to teach the concept of humor.

---

## Advantages

- A cartoon makes its point instantaneously.
- It has emotional impact.
- It is often esthetically pleasing.
- It promotes critical thinking.
- It is easy to read.
- It is exciting.
- It satisfies an unsophisticated idea of art.
- It is a versatile, inexpensive, contemporary tool for the teacher.
- It is increasingly being used in education as well as nursing.

## Disadvantages

- A cartoon employs stereotypes that may have lost meaning.
- It may be culturally biased.
- It is quite abstract and depends on rather full background for correct interpretations.
- On controversial subjects it is one-sided and biased.
- It may oversimplify -- and oversimplification may give false impressions.
- It has debatable value in education -- some consider it childish.

---

## Points to Remember

- Use skillfully and judiciously.
- Relate it to the subject so that learners can interpret implications correctly.
- Because of use of stereotypes, teacher must accompany cartoon with emphasis on the dynamic, changing nature of reality

- Research (done in 1960) indicates that generally the earliest age at which children can make correct interpretations of exaggerated drawings is 13 year.
- Discussion is generally essential.
- Students may draw their own cartoons and write as well as talk about their interpretations.
- Students may need to be taught a critical approach to the cartoon as well as the topic.
- Cartoons may be used on bulletin board, chalkboard, as handouts, or projected (opaque, overhead, or a 2-by-2-inch slide).
- The teacher may find it helpful to collect and file cartoons.

**References**

Block, A., & Brooks, M. (1978). Cartoons for cardiology artistry and articulation. Biomedical Communications, 6 (4), 16-20.

Culhane, J. (1979). The funnies are us. Readers Digest, 115 (688), 163-170.

Dale, E. (1969). Audiovisual methods in teaching, (3rd ed., pp. 512-515). New York: Dryden Press, Holt, Rinehart & Winston. (Basic content on this method.)

Hatfield, P. (1976). Come on, Charlie Brown, let's go play. American Journal of Nursing 76 (10), 1611-1612. (The author uses a cartoon to introduce selected nursing concepts.)

Kinder, J. S. (1973). Using instructional media. (pp. 92-94.) New York: D. Van Nostrand. (Briefly discusses the value and use of cartoons and comics.)

Nelson, R. P. (1975). Cartooning. Chicago: Henry Regency. (A history of cartooning that gives suggestions for creating cartoons.)

Pease, R. (1991). Cartoon humor in nursing education. Nursing Outlook, 39, 262-267.

Robinson, V. M. (1977). Humor and the health professions. Thorofare, NJ: C.B. Slack. (A recent book on humor that does not speak directly about cartoons although each chapter contains cartoons.)

Weaver, W. T. (1970). Humor and education. Phi Delta Kappan, 70(3), 166-168. (An educator and cartoonist writes a historical review of cartoons in education.)

Rana, I. (1987). Comics-for health. Development Communication Report, 4 (59), 1-3.

## CASE STUDY

### Definition

*Case Study* is an account of a problem situation, including enough detail for learners to suggest possible solutions.

### Purposes

- Lend reality to indirect experience.
- Increase interest and involvement in learning.
- Think independently and cooperatively.
- Give synthesis and meaning to separate parts of the whole, interrelating knowledge.
- Develop skill in decision-making and problem-solving.
- Pool the insights of group members.
- Broaden experience.
- Bridge the gap between theory and practice.
- Analyze motives and issues in the affective domain.
- Focus on concrete situations and examples.
- Help learners see problems in proper perspective.
- Assist the learner to see a problem from many points of view.
- Demonstrate that few hard questions have easy answers.
- Help learners avoid "causal oversimplification."

---

**Advantages**

- Interest and "appeal."
- Realism and "life likeness."
- Provide for examples of specific and concrete problems.
- Interrelate knowledge, parts and whole.
- Develop decision making and problem solving skills.

**Disadvantages**

- Validity of the method is directly related to the reality of the case.
- Assumes readiness of learner; factual and maturational.
- May be tendency to oversimplify.
- Takes time to become acquainted with the method -- both learner and teacher.
- Requires time for teacher to prepare the case and to prepare own role when it is used in the classroom.

---

## Forms

- Classical case study -- a rather comprehensive record of the various kinds of evidence that bear upon a problem. Includes such information as: biographical data, psychological evidence, social evidences, economic considerations, relational evidences, historical data, statistical information, biological-pathological data, etc. The case may or may not be written.
- Unfinished story -- usually ends with "What should you do?" (An example of this is found as a monthly feature in the journal for teachers, Today's Education.)
- Embryo case -- just enough information is presented to establish a problem
- Critical incident case -- confronts the learner at the explosion point in a problem. Best described as a "now-that-it-has-happened-what-do-I-do?"
- Report analysis case -- invites learners to study data in reports of various kinds.
- Cartoon teaser case -- permits learners to fill in answers to problems presented by cartoon characters.
- Informational "what-do-you-see?" case -- serves as a stimulus to recall information about persons, places, things, or events. A picture may be used.
- Psychological "what-do-you-see?" case -- asks the learner to analyze a picture in light of psychological factors involved. May be effective in considering cultural diversity.
- "In-basket" case -- the learner makes decisions based on the nature of the correspondence. Policy and procedure may help or hinder the decision-making.
- Impromptu case -- emphasis is on the dynamics of the present situation. Teacher may call attention to incidents which develop in the group and use them as cases.
- "Ex post facto" case -- evaluation of a decision already made. "Did-I-act-wisely?"
- "Baited" case -- when significant parts are deliberately withheld. Learners learn to search further, weed out the unimportant, and delete the insignificant material.
- Educational simulation case -- permits learners to act out their responses to direct, made-up experiences.

## Format

- Discover or define the problem, source of conflicts or confusion.
- Define the basic issues.
- Discuss the problem (determine possible solutions and the best solutions).
- Dissolve the problem (take action, if appropriate).

## Responsibilities

1. Learner:
   a. Be willing to share ideas and information.
   b. Prepare ahead of time, whether written case is provided or not.
   c. Follow the steps in methodology (or modify within the group).

2. Teacher:
   a. Establish a non authoritarian atmosphere in which the learners are very free to speak in an uninhibited way.
   b. Prepare before hand for primary role -- probably not gathering a lot of data which is the learner's responsibility to contribute.
   c. Primary function during discussion: keep track of learner's comments and be prepared at any time to summarize, point out dilemmas, and ask for relevancy or evidence.
   d. Prepare the case study (either written or not), or select one consistent with objectives.

**Sources of Case Studies**

- Personal experiences of learners or teachers.
- Comments overheard in "everyday life."
- Professional journals.
- Textbooks, pamphlets.
- Biographies, autobiographies, fiction, lay publications.
- Newspapers -- news items, "advice columns," cartoons.
- Resource people and other experts may be requested to provide them.

**Combined with other Methods**

Brainstorming -- may be especially useful if the case is being studied by a large group and small groups are used to determine solutions.
Printed case history -- the printed material of the case is written in advance; permitting advance and post-discussion study.
Debate -- group members debate the pros and cons of a suggested solution.
Symposium -- a symposium of experts present their analyses of the case. (This then becomes a part of the case.)
Listening teams -- groups listen according to predetermined assignments.
Audio and video tape replays -- may add reality and/or clarity to the case.
Films -- using a case presented via films; stopping at various points for discussion and perhaps not showing the entire film.
Role-playing -- may help members identify more readily with a problem. May be used at various times in the case.

**References**

Andrews, K. R. (1956). The case method of teaching human relations and administration Cambridge, MA: Harvard University Press. (An old, classic source.)

Cooper, R. M. (1958). The two ends of the log (pp. 238-241). Minneapolis, MN: University of Minnesota Press. (A brief discussion of the method in teaching.)

Cooper, S. (1981). Methods of teaching -- revisited, case method. Journal of Continuing Education in Nursing, 12 (5), 32-36.

Dailey, M. (1992). Developing case studies. Nurse Educator, 17, 8-11.

Ford, L. (1969). Using the case study in teaching and training Nashville, TN: Broadman Press. (A book of cartoons featuring the use of the method. Intended for religious education; delightful to read.)

Johnson, J. (1987). Case studies: An alternative learning/teaching method in nursing. Journal of Nursing Education, 26, 118-120.

McNair, M. (Ed.). (1954). The case method at the harvard business school. New York: McGraw-Hill. (Another classic in the use of this method in the early '50s.)

Mitchell, C. A., & Ayello, E. A. (1976). Hygiene made interesting: The case method. Journal of Nursing Education, 15 (5), 11-13.

Mitchell, J., Jr. (1981). The use of case studies in bioethics courses. Journal of Nursing Education, 20 (9), 31-36.

O'Connell, A., & Bates, B. (1976). The case method in nursing practitioner education. Nursing Outlook, 24 (4), 243-246.

# CHALKBOARD

## Definition

*Chalkboard* is a board whose writing surface is especially treated to use with chalk.
Synonym -- Blackboard

## Purposes

- Illustrates facts, ideas, and processes.
- Clarifies concepts with the help of drawings, sketches, maps, and diagrams.
- Presents important facts and principles (new words, definitions, classifications).
- Demonstrates students' ideas.
- Displays a wide variety of methods.
- Displays the decorative and creative work of learners.
- Assists both the teacher and learners in impromptu presentations.
- Attracts and holds attention.

## Advantages

- Cost is minimal.
- A chalkboard is usually available -- a portable chalkboard may be used when a permanent one is not at hand.
- It requires little practice and equipment.
- It permits on-the-spot revision.
- It is a versatile medium.
- It adds interest and variety for learners.
- Teacher may incorporate learners' ideas at the time they are suggested.
- A chalkboard may supplement or complement other teaching methods (demonstrations, maps).
- It is useful for all age groups.
- Visual information can be added progressively.

## Disadvantages

- A chalkboard does not provide a permanent record.
- It has limited use in large groups and cannot show intricate detail.
- It may be overused, improperly used, and/or considered unimportant as a method.
- Teacher may fail to use it creatively (or carefully).
- It is confusing to the learner if too much information is presented.

## Combined Forms

1. Chalkboards and demonstrations
   a. Stages or steps in a process can be outlined.
   b. It is available throughout the demonstration.
   c. It allows important parts of the demonstration to be sketched quickly.

**Points to Remember**

- Keep chalkboard clean.
- Erase thoroughly before and during use.
- Print and draw large and neatly.
- Check for glare.
- Avoid obscuring the board.
- If content (problem or drawing) is complex, put all or part on board before presentation.
- If material is too complex, select another method, such as a handout.
- Avoid crowding the board.
- Avoid unnecessary details.
- Practice, try new ways (including colored chalk, permanent chalk).
- Use creative forms when appropriate:
  a. Disclosure method
     (1) Hidden chalkboard-cover the work on the board with a poster board until ready to use.
     (2) Strip chart -- fasten strips of paper to the chalkboard until ready to use.
  b. Embellished chart -- use a movable pointer attached with adhesive.
  c. Permanent aid -- paint designs on board as permanent background (for forms used often in teaching).
  d. Drawings traced from opaque projector -- maps and designs may be traced on the board from an opaque projector.
- Combine with cork board, pegboard, or other boards.
- Erase well after use -- a habit guaranteed to make colleagues happy.
- Stabilize a portable board before using it.
- Guest speakers may wish to be sure of a chalkboard by bringing a portable, collapsible chalkboard (and chalk!).
- Semi-permanent chalk is useful for drawings or information you wish retained from one period to another. Recipe for semi-permanent chalk:
  a. Prepare a saturated sugar solution by stirring sufficient sugar into a cup of cold water so that after vigorous shaking or stirring a small amount of sugar still remains in the bottom of the container. Prepare a second solution consisting of one part of the sugar solution to three parts of cold water. Soak a few sticks of regular chalk in this solution. When the chalk no longer effervesces (5-10 minutes), remove chalk and drain for short time on paper toweling.
  b. Treated chalk can be stored indefinitely in a closed container.
  c. Remove lines made with this chalk with a damp cloth.

**Other Related Methodologies:** Flipchart

## References


Dale, E. (1969). Audiovisual methods in teaching (3rd ed., pp. 287-291). New York: Dryden Press, Holt, Rinehart & Winston. (A classic source of information.)

Day, R. S. (1967). The original teaching machine -- the blackboard. Educational Forum, 31 (2), 195-200. (Gives the history of the chalkboard.)

Ford, L. (1963). A primer for teachers and leaders (p. 109). Nashville, TN: Broadman Press. (Presents uses of the chalkboard in cartoon form.)

Glattbach, J. (1978). Erasable print -- blackboard newspapers. Development Communication Report, 21, 6-7.

Gustafson, M. B. (1977). The blackboard chalkboard revisited. Supervisor Nurse, 8 (5), 57-58. (Includes much of the content in this guideline, but in greater detail.)

Morgan, B., Holmes, G. E., & Bundy, C. E. (1976). Methods in adult education (3rd ed., p. 199). Danville, IL: Interstate Printers & Publishers. (Discusses use of the chalkboard with adults.)

# CHART

**Definition**

*Chart* is a generic term for any systematic arrangement of facts in graphic or pictorial form, presenting for convenient reference comparisons of quality, distributions, trends, summaries, etc.

**Purposes**

- To visualize an idea or concept that would be difficult to understand if treated only verbally.
- To present material clearly and concisely.
- To provide an outline of materials covered in a presentation.
- To highlight important points.

---

**Advantages**

- Reduce the amount of verbal explanation necessary to understand interrelationships and specific information.
- Illustrate a single fact or concept or a sequence.
- Inexpensive to prepare (from cheap paper or cardboard).
- Reusable.
- Useful for a wide range of learners and variety of settings.
- Useful at a variety of points-overview, as an outline, or summary.
- Use an intermixture of visual materials-pictures, drawings, cartoons, graphs, diagrams.
- May be combined with other tools-both projected and non-projected (chalkboard, transparencies, slides, posters).

**Disadvantages**

- Requires thoughtful planning and time to select and/or prepare.
- Teacher needs to review, update, and modify original charts.
- Learners need to know how to "read" charts.
- Commercial ones may be expensive and require storage space.
- May not be appropriate to size of group, size of room or to use.

---

**Types of Charts:** (There are various classification systems).

- Experience charts -- records of stories, news, and experiences.
- Organization charts -- flow charts, stream charts, tree charts, tabular charts, process charts.
- Time charts -- chronology, historical events.
- Other -- map, pictorial, issue.

**Points to Remember**

- Construct or select based on objectives and criteria.
- Digest material and be sure you are familiar with the major points and their implications.

- Choose most important points to illustrate on chart -- Don't have too much detail or too many concepts.
- If using more than one chart, concern for sequence.
- In developing, plan for legibility, lettering, proper size and related graphics.
- May project (overhead), enlarge (wall chart), make poster, etc., to accompany small copies given to individual learners for their personal use.
- Place chart at proper height. Check for glare.
- Glance at chart only briefly.
- Don't block view of chart, use pointer for emphasis.

**Other Related Methodologies:** Model, Graphics, Flow Chart, Diagrams, Graphs, Posters, Cartoons, Comics.

**References**


Dale, E. Audiovisual methods in teaching (3rd ed., pp. 522-525). New York: Dryden Press, Holt, Rinehart & Winston.

Kinder, J. S. Using instructional media (pp. 105-108). New York: D. Van Nost & Co.

Morgan, B., Holmes, C. E., & Bundy, C. E. (1976). Methods in adult education (3rd ed., pp. 200-201). Danville, IL: Interstate Printers & Publishers.

Santos, C. G., & Setty, L. R. (1975). Charts and models from cardboard. Biomedical Communications, 3 (2), 14-15. (Medical school professors discuss use of large wall to floor size charts and models made from corrugated cardboard.)

# CINQUAIN

## Definition

*Cinquain* is a five line stanza.

## Purposes

- Stimulates new thoughts about an old idea.
- Demonstrates creativity.
- Teaches an English poetry form.

---

**Advantages**

- Composition involves learner in the development of creativity.
- It requires little time and orientation, and yields much.
- No special equipment is needed.

---

## Procedure

- Title -- a noun.
- Two words that describe -- adjectives.
- Three words that express action -- verbs.
- Four words that express feeling.
- Title -- repeated or a synonym.

**Sample of Cinquain** (one that doesn't meet the specifications above):

ANGUISH

Keep thou
Thy tearless watch
All night. When blue dawn
Breathes on the silver moon, then weep.
Then weep!

-Adelaide Crapsey

## References


Burnside, I. M. (1970). Cinquains for my aged patients. American Journal of Nursing 70 (11), 2357. (A nurse presents examples of cinquains.)

Crapsey, A. (1926). Verse. New York: Alfred A Knopf. (A book of poems by the American writer who originated cinquains.)

# CLIP ART

## Definition

*Clip Art* is a line and tone ready-to-use illustrations prepared commercially, covering a wide variety of subject classifications.

## Purposes

- Add interest and attention to a variety of visuals being prepared -- transparencies, posters, newsletters, brochures, worksheets, etc.
- Provide visual materials for those without drawing skill or when it is necessary to repeat symbols.
- Assist teachers in producing visual materials with a professional appearance.

---

## Advantages

- Assist non-artistic individuals in preparing materials.
- Saves time in preparing materials when symbols or other repetitive silhouette visuals are needed.
- Inexpensive.
- Generally removes copyright concerns in use of drawings.
- May be combined with lettering and graphs.

## Disadvantages

- Some subjects are more difficult to obtain than others.
- Drawings may still need to be enlarged or reduced.
- Collection and storage may be a problem.

---

## Points to Remember

- Clip art should clarify concepts or ideas, not confuse.
- May wish to subscribe to receive commercially updated or newly designed clip art sheets or books periodically.
- Personal file may include any materials that would be useful as clip art -- providing copyright is observed.

## References


Gustafson, M. (1987). Teaching tips: Clip art. Journal of Continuing Education in Nursing, 18 139.

Kemp, J. E. (1975). Planning and producing audiovisual materials (3rd ed.).

Minor, E. (1978). Handbook for preparing visual media (2nd ed., p. 38). New York: McGraw-Hill. (Lists clip art sources.)

Minor, E., & Frye, H. R. (1970). Techniques for producing visual instructional media (pp. 30-31). New York; McGraw-Hill. (Discusses uses and sources.)

# COLLAGE

## Definition

*Collage* refers to sticking things together on a board. It is an art form which has become popular and increasingly significant. Early use followed the development of paper when Japanese used it in ornamentation of text, and later used by artists like Picasso, Braque, and Schwitters.

## Purposes

- Take already existing things and arrange according to an idea or feeling.
- Look at things around you in a new way.
- Express emotions -- both by the visual, and when discussed.
- Provide group work as an interactive teaching strategy.
- Stimulate discussion and reflection.

---

**Advantages**

- Uses actual shapes and surfaces of ordinary things from real life.
- Explore abstract design with a wide range of pictorial or descriptive subjects.
- Can be enjoyed by everyone.
- May be made very inexpensively (from scraps, odds and ends).
- Can be as simple or elaborate as desired.
- Share expressive possibilities of an individual or group.

**Disadvantages**

- May be seen as play
- Requires some work space and collection of materials.

---

## Materials Needed (3 basic areas)

Support surface: paper, cardboard, or various boards of wood, such as half inch plywood.
Objects to be placed on the surface: paper, cloth, memorabilia, collections, or mixed media.
Adhesive: glue, gum, paste, spray mount.

## Points to Remember

- Where you place the first piece of paper (or other object) will decide the character of the final work.
- You may wish to read standard texts on materials in each of the three basic areas.
- Seymour suggests you provide guidelines for preparation and for discussion and reflection.

**References**


Borja, C., & Borja, R. (1972). Making collages. Chicago: Albert Whitman & Co.

Digby, J., & Digby, J. (1985). The collage handbook. New York: Thames & Hudson.

Portchmouth, J. (1995). Working in collage. New York: The Viking Press.

Seymour, R. (1995). Creating a collage: A meaningful interactive classroom strategy. Nurse Educator, 20 (3), 19-21.

# COLLOQUY

## Definition

*Colloquy* is a method of collective inquiry characterized by the presentation of testimony by a group of experts, and questions, answers, and discussion by both the experts and the audience on the matter under consideration.

## Purposes

- Stimulates interest in a topic.
- Identifies, clarifies, or solves problems.
- Identifies and explores issues.
- Brings expert knowledge to bear on problems as they emerge from discussion.
- Gives the audience opportunities to understand the component parts of a topic.
- Weights the advantages and disadvantages of a course of action.
- Reduces the natural barriers that usually stand between a large audience and resource persons, thus helping to establish rapport between audience and experts.
- Offers resource persons the opportunity to get a clear picture of the audience's knowledge of the topic.

---

## Advantages

- In a colloquy, a large audience can be represented, with some opportunity for direct participation.
- Audience representatives can get clarification if a vague or abstract statement is made by the resource person.
- The audience members are encouraged to feel responsibility for their representatives and therefore to listen and participate actively.
- The method reduces natural barriers between audience and resource person.
- Since moderator guides discussion toward topics of concern as they emerge, colloquy permits considerable flexibility in the learning situation.
- Resource persons tend to consider carefully the problems and needs of the audience.

## Disadvantages

- Experienced moderators of colloquy are not always available.
- Audience members may be hesitant to participate actively.
- Audience and its representatives may not be sufficiently informed to ask meaningful questions of resource persons.
- Resource persons are not always willing to listen to questions and make their remarks relatively brief and to the point.
- Because of limited time, it may not always be fully explored, and defended.

---

## Format and Persons Involved

- ➢ Moderator. Guides the discussion of the resource persons, the audience representatives, and the audience. He or she is skilled in the use of techniques of discussion and in stimulating participation by a large audience.
- ➢ Resource persons. Usually one to four persons chosen for their particular knowledge and interest in the subject to be discussed, and their ability to participate in an informal manner.
- ➢ Audience representatives. Chosen for their interest in the topic and ability to ask questions and make intelligent comments so as to clarify ideas for themselves and the audience. They are chosen in advance by a planning committee or during the meeting.
- ➢ Audience. Usually composed of persons interested in the topic.

**Responsibilities of Members**

- Moderator
  - a. Prior to colloquy
    1. Plans for physical setup that will aid informal discussion and problem solving.
    2. Has clearly in mind the topics and desired goals.
    3. Assesses the characteristics of the group anticipated. Considers these in orienting the resource persons.
    4. Determines point in discussion when audience is invited to participate verbally.
    5. Plans and carries out steps to encourage advanced reading and follow-up study.
    6. Gets acquainted with resource persons and audience representatives and informs them of topics to be covered, goals to be reached, characteristics of the group, and other mechanics.
    7. Plans the introduction.
  - b. During the colloquy
    1. Presents introduction.
    2. Encourages and develops audience participation, at time decided.
    3. Restates and clearly directs questions from audience representatives and audience; refrains from entering into the discussion and answering questions.
    4. Tries to develop and maintain friendly, informal atmosphere.
    5. Recognizes members of audience one at a time.
    6. Directs course of discussion to fit situations that arise.
    7. Remains neutral if controversy arises.
    8. Tries to prevent a monopoly of discussion by one person or a few.
    9. Summarizes when necessary.
    10. Allows appropriate amount of time for each topic.
    11. Prevents resource persons from dominating the discussion.
    12. Suggests follow-up study by all participants if advisable.
- Resource persons.
  - a. Prior to colloquy
    1. Familiarize themselves with the colloquy technique.
    2. Prepare to participate informally
    3. Prepare to talk about topics that are likely to emerge.
    4. Study characteristics of the group and the relationship of colloquy to total program, if appropriate.

b. During the colloquy
   1. Contribute when their opinions are needed -- in language the audience understands.
   2. Make brief, direct comments appropriate to the questions asked.
   3. Refrain from using the occasion to promote ideas not directly applicable.
   4. Avoid disparaging remarks about contributions of audience and its representatives.
   5. Encourage audience participation.

- Audience representatives
  a. Prior to colloquy
     1. Inform themselves about purpose, goals, and topics.
     2. Develop questions and comments to put to resource persons.
  b. During the colloquy
     1. Present topics to resource persons in form of comments, problems, and questions.
     2. Ask for clarification and explanation.
     3. Attempt to make their contributions clear and to the point.
     4. Show interest and seek to stimulate audience participation.
- Audience members
  a. Study and prepare in advance.
  b. Listen thoughtfully and participate verbally when called for.
  c. Support and encourage their representatives.
  d. Insist that all persons deal with the concerns of the audience.

**Suggestions for Use**

- Select a moderator carefully, since much success depends on his or her efficiency.
- Be prepared for variety in original interest, intelligence levels, knowledge, and information about the topic.
- Adapt program to audience needs and interests.
- Make necessary arrangements for physical setup.
- Check out public address system if necessary.
- Use comfortable seating arrangement, and name cards (big enough for audience to read easily).
- See guidelines for "guest speaker" for some aspects of planning.
- Make sure all participants are familiar with the method.

**Other Related Methodologies:** Panel

**References**

Bergevin, P., Morris, D., & Smith, R. (1963). Adult education procedures (pp. 42-54). New York: Seabury Press. (A very useful book with much detail.)

Cooper, S. (1979). Methods of teaching -- Revisited: Colloquy. Journal of Continuing Education in Nursing, 10 (2), 36-38.

Morgan, H., Holmes, G., & Bundy, C. (1976). Methods in adult education (3rd ed., p. 83). Danville, IL: Interstate Printers & Publishers, Inc.

# COLOR

**Definition**

*Color* is a stylistic convention of visual representation and an attribute.

**Purposes**

- Heighten realism, approximate original, show what something is naturally like.
- Emphasize, distinguish and see differences.
- Produce significant effect on emotions (aesthetic and psychological effects).
- Color can draw attention and place emphasis where needed.

---

**Advantages**

- Important to learning process.
- Add appeal, interest, and attention getting.
- Meaning and preferences are culturally determined.
- Color has carrying, magical power.
- Can be culture specific when assessment is done.

**Disadvantages**

- Culture determines meaning and preferences.
- Need to know recent research.
- Value and power may be assumed and not utilized.

---

**Points to Remember**

- Add color if it's important to your educational/informational intentions.
- Utilize cross-cultural research for maximum value with cultural groups (ethnic groups, subcultures).
- Make color work by planning, since neither use nor failure to use should be simply habitual or unplanned.
- Knowledge of color wheel may be helpful -- such as concepts of harmony in combining colors:
    - monochromatic -- shades of one color
    - analogous -- neighbors on wheel
    - complementary -- opposites on wheel
- May wish to include knowledge of preference and those with positive association.
- Seek information regarding contrast when working with layout, background, lettering, etc., for construction of visuals (i.e., booklets, posters, bulletin boards).
- Pretest colored materials in cross-cultural settings.

## Selected Factors From Cross-cultural Research

- There are focal colors that are more easily perceived by all human beings: 11 basic colors (represented in English) by 8 chromatic -- red, yellow, green, brown, blue, orange, pink and purple; 3 achromatic -- black, white, gray.
- Physiological factors might influence development of color terms rather than language culturally determining color perceptions.
- Many languages sparse color terminology, but not an inability to perceive color (i.e., leaf-colored).
- Culture mediates our learning processes so pervasively that it remains experimentally impossible to conclusively separate perceptual influences that are purely physiological from ones that are purely cultural.
- Issue of ability to discriminate is not apt to be involved in differences in terminology from culture to culture, since man can discriminate 7,500,000 colors (but no language names more than a few).
- Perhaps color coding is more easily and rapidly learned in cultures possessing a rich repertoire of distinct color terms.
- If color is intended to communicate information in cultural contexts different from originally designed (and especially those with no formal education), it may fail to transmit intended message.

## References


Dale, E. (1969). Audiovisual methods in teaching (3rd ed.). New York: Dryden Press.

Kwansa, E., et al. (1972). Perception and comprehension of health education visual aids by rural Ghanian villagers. Ghana Medical Journal, 11, 387-396.

Mangan, J. (1978). Cultural conventions of pictorial representation: Iconic literacy and education. Educational Communication and Technology Journal, 26, 259-261.

Minor, E. (1978). Handbook for preparing visual media. New York: McGraw-Hill.

Pett, D. (N.D.). Audiovisual communication handbook. Oklahoma City, OK: World Neighbors.

# CONFERENCE

## Definition

*Conference* is a meeting of two or more persons of common interest who come together to consider a particular subject, or for consultation, discussion and interchange of opinions and ideas.

## Purposes

- Provide for productive interchange of ideas and opinions.
- Provide for a group to consider a topic or subject.

---

**Advantages**

- Bring people together from different geographic areas and backgrounds.
- Provide study and sharing away from usual work setting.
- The cost of bringing in experts is shared by the group.
- Individual can gain insights from others to broaden perspective.

**Disadvantages**

- May be expensive.
- Requires much planning and organizing.
- If held at a distance from home, may involve time in travel and housing arrangements.
- Assessment of learner is difficult.

---

## Primary Aspects to Consider

- Planning.
- Attending (selection and preparation of participants).
- Reporting and recording.

## Suggestions for Planners

- Probably need a checklist and helps for planning a successful meeting.
- Depending on the size and location, there are a variety of aspects to consider.
- Begin with objectives and planning committee.
- Establish timetable, delegate responsibilities, determine cost and begin publicity.
- Decide on methods to be used and time committed.
- Decide on individuals to present, speak, lead.
- Determine needs for facilities, equipment, schedule and tasks to be assigned.
- Assign tasks as appropriate.

**Attendance** (Individual or agency responsibility to determine)

- Determine if, who, and why, one will attend.
- If more than one individual is attending, should preplanning be done to determine if a variety of options should be sampled.
- Determine if it is necessary to report back to sending agency and in what form. (Written, oral, forms).

**Other Related Methodologies:** Guest Speakers, Exhibits, Displays, Panel, Lecture, Seminar, Meeting, Workshop.

**References**


Cooper, S. S. (1976). Getting the most out of a conference. Journal of Continuing Education in Nursing, 7 (5), 11-17. (Specific suggestions for participants.)

Finkel, C. (1978). Professional guide to successful meetings. Madison, WI: American Society for Training and Development. (May be a useful guide book for planners.)

Hoyt, J. S., Jr. (1977). Personal time management and effective administration (6th ed.). Minneapolis, MN: University of Minnesota Agricultural Extension Services. (Contains excellent lengthy checklists with areas to note who is responsible and the timetable.)

Lewis, E. (1976, November). The meeting season. [Editorial]. Nursing Outlook, 24 (11), 675. (Briefly and humorously points out some things that result from attending meetings.)

McCone, A. (1971). Sending someone to a conference? Here are some tips. Canadian Nurse, 67 (2), 36-37. (Brief article follows the stated title in content.)

Medearis, N. D. (1973, January/February). You can help it happen. [Editorial]. Journal of Nursing Administration, 3 (1), 12-13. (Expectations of those who attend meetings are discussed from point of view of one who conducts meetings.)

## CONTEST

**Definition**

*Contest* is an organized competition where performance of specific works are compared (as to merit) and judged.

**Purpose**

- Competition of creative activity for rating of merit based on standards. The awarding of prizes may be involved.

---

**Advantages**

- Increase involvement and interest.
- Stimulate creativity intrinsically and motivation externally.
- Reward meritorious work.
- May be simple or elaborate, inexpensive or expensive.
- May be individual or group.

**Disadvantages**

- Competition in some cultures may be unusual and undesirable.

---

**Possible Contests:**

Development of a song or slogan.
Poster development (health fair, poster session.)
Preparation of materials for staff development.

**Points to Remember**

- Contestants need to know the established rules and guidelines as to use of materials, amount to spend, and size (as of posters). You may wish to provide entry blanks and some materials.
- Clearly set dates and places where projects are due.
- Provide information about judging -- such as the criteria for judging and who are the judges (peers, students, the general public, experts).
- Indicate what the award or prize will be. Additional prize ideas: a book (pertinent to your discipline) or certificate of membership (to a spa). It is possible some business with which you are affiliated may wish to contribute as item as a prize. As with other aspects of contests, prizes do not have to be lavish, but a cash prize is often considered special.
- Notification and publication of winners may occur in a newsletter or an in-house publication or may occur at a scheduled event complete with certificate and a celebration of some kind.

## References

(1991). CFNI. Nutrition 'Song Contest' a hit in Jamaica. Cajanus, 24 (2), 113-114.

Petersen, J. (1994). Increasing standards awareness through a Fortune Cookie Contest. Journal of Continuing Education in Nursing, 25 (1), 48.

Modic, M. & Harris, R. (1994). A reinforcement technique: The goody bag. Journal of Continuing Education in Nursing, 25 (3), 143-144.

Ribeiro, M. (1989). AIDS Song contest in Guinea-Bissau. World Health Forum, 10, 107-108.

Silayan-Go, A. (1990). Entertainment for health. World Health Forum, 11, 297-301.

# CONTRADICTION

## Definition

*Contradiction* is one of the forms of conceptual conflict used to stimulate curiosity by successively presenting opposing facts on a topic and demanding explanations.

## Purposes

- A provocative way of present ideas.
- Provides another form of discovery learning.

---

**Advantages**

- Relatively unrestricted to subject matter or level limitations.
- Basically simple, yet interesting.
- Requires little orientation.
- Sharpens students awareness of ideas involved in the contradiction.
- Points out that there are many possible explanation.

**Disadvantages**

- Need to provide requisite information if it's available.

---

## Points to Remember

- Prepare to orient learners to format.
- Need for two sets of facts that constitute the contradiction (usually order is not important).
- Both sets of facts must be credible.
- Material must be appropriate to level of learner (neither too easy nor too difficult). Must challenge.
- Answer has to be provided, conflict has to be resolved.

## Example

An example might be a change in nursing action as the result of new research finding.

## References

Berlyn, D. (1965). Curiosity and education. In J. Krumbotty (Ed.), Learning and the educational process. Chicago: Rand McNally.

Vidler, D. (1974). The use of contradiction to stimulate curiosity. Educational technology, 14 (10), 41-43

# CRITIQUE HOUR

## Definition

*Critique Hour* is a class session providing students with the opportunity to critique.
*Critique* -- 1) criticism or critical examination, 2) scholarly analysis of an essay, article or other work, 3) a critical estimate of an activity designed primarily for the purpose of improving one's future performance therein, 4) review of work with a student to point out his/her strong and weak points in practice and offer suggestions for improvement. (Good)

## Purposes

- To develop the skill of analyzing the strengths and weakness of ideas and plans as objectively as possible.
- To identify the strengths and weakness of ideas and plans as objectively as possible.
- To provide a forum for the interchange of ideas among students.
- To suggest alternative, creative approaches to teaching.
- To introduce the student to peer learning, peer teaching, and peer review.

---

## Advantages

- Increased ability to look at your own and others' ideas and plans objectively.
- Provide peer group input into an individual's lesson plan.
- Provide students the opportunity to gain a respect for each other's attitudes, philosophies, creativity, and other attributes.
- Provide for students to build or "hitchhike" on ideas originated/generated by a peer.
- Provide an opportunity to share materials and media.
- Critique class session may be used to actually experience or use material, i.e., pretest an assessment tool, review a peer-made audio-tape.
- Improved product as the result of multiple input.

## Disadvantages

- Could become destructive rather than constructive if entire focus is negative criticism.
- May result in "show and tell" session if analysis is not built in.

---

## Responsibilities of Group Members

- Mutual trust needs to be developed.
- The teacher is generally a member of the group and has the same responsibilities.
- Some form of written material (i.e., lesson plan, tool) may save repeated explanations if prepared ahead of the session and shared in writing (and/or distributed prior to the hour).

- Group members need to view the criticism as assistance and both give and take in the critique hour.
- Some pre-scheduling for specific sharing or bringing of plans may facilitate optimum use of the class hour.
- At end of session, or periodically, may want to add an analysis of the group's ability to critique.

**Other Related Methodologies:** Self Examination, Critical Thinking, Exchange Of Ideas, Public Speaking Critique, Learning-to-Listen Critique,

**References**


Bergevin, P., Morris, D., & Smith, R. M. (1963). Adult education procedures. New York: Seabury Press. (Contains brief descriptions of sub techniques.)

Good, C. V. (1973). Dictionary of education (3rd ed.). New York: McGraw-Hill.

Satinsky, V. P. (1974). Critiques as an instrument for education. The Science Teacher, 41 (4), 28-29. (A high school teacher suggests the method with high ability students.)

## Definition

*Debate* is a persuasive activity. A parliamentary procedure designed to give proponents and opponents of a measure as nearly equal opportunities as possible to present their evidence and to argue their conclusions before a group who will make a decision.

## Purposes

- Arouse interest in a problem.
- Practice in analyzing current problems.
- Improve critical thinking ability.
- Defend a thesis against attack.
- Foster "thinking on one's feet" -- verbalize thoughts extemporaneously.
- Learn the value of speaking when something is at stake.
- Provide a way to gain self-confidence.
- Enable one to learn to be tolerant of differing views.
- Design concise cogent arguments that can stand up under attack.
- Identify fallacious arguments.

---

**Advantages**

- Promotes looking at two extreme sides of an issue.
- Separates the pros and cons of an issue or solution.
- Requires logical support of ideas.
- Provides time limits and a decision, unlike bull sessions where arguments may go on endlessly.
- Faculty and/or learners may be the debaters.

**Disadvantages**

- May deepen disagreements.
- May heighten emotional tension.
- Debaters may be identified with a position to which they've been assigned rather than one they accept.
- Not appropriate when listeners are just beginning to learn about a problem; such situations call for exposition and analysis, not argument.
- Not helpful during time of crisis.

---

## Essential Characteristics

- The debater begins with a judgment which he/she urges others to accept or to reject. The judgment may be about facts, values, or policies.
- The judgment must be so stated in the form of a motion, resolution, bill, proposition or indictment as to give the voter a choice between two alternatives. The judgment is stated in a form that requires the affirmative team to suggest a change in the present system. Both sides have an equal opportunity to present their arguments, following a schedule which

alternates arguments for and against the motion and allowing each side the same number of minutes. The burden of proof rests on the affirmative.

- When the allotted time has expired, a vote is taken and the will of the majority is the decision.

**<u>Format for Formal Debate</u>**

<u>Constructive Speeches</u> (10 minutes each)
First affirmative
First negative
Second affirmative
Second negative

<u>Rebuttals</u> (5 minutes each)
First negative
First affirmative
Second negative
Second affirmative

**<u>Procedure</u>**

- Building the "Case"
  The case is a series of statements which, if supported to the satisfaction of the listener, should logically lead them to the desired conclusion. The statements should present the strongest arguments found in constructing the argument.
- General Rules for Building the Case
  a. Statements should be arranged to show a progression of ideas; the strongest argument should be presented early in the debate.
  b. Main points should be few in number; three or four fundamental propositions, well supported by evidence.
  c. Relations between statements should be clearly indicated.
  d. Phrasing of the statements should have "headline value"; phrased in short sentences and everyday words.
  e. Case should not attempt to prove too much. Debate should be an exercise in restraint and discrimination.
- General Outline of:
  A. Affirmative Speeches
    1.) First Affirmative Speech
      a.) Introduction
        i.) show why question is of interest and importance.
        ii.) give explanation and historical background as necessary.
        iii.) careful definition of terms.
        iv.) state main issues and give main points in the case, containing answers to these issues.
      b.) Discussion
        i.) state main points and support with evidence.

ii.) clearly indicate relation of each point.

c.) Conclusion

i.) summarize argument.

ii.) show progress toward proving case.

2.) Second Affirmative Speech

a.) Introduction

i.) briefly analyze the first negative speech.

ii.) restate main affirmative contentions.

iii.) summarize first affirmative speech.

b.) Discussion

i.) present and support main contentions.

c.) Conclusion

i.) summarize argument and progress.

b. The Negative Case

1.) First Negative Speech

a.) Introduction

i.) accept or reject the affirmative analysis and definitions.

ii.) refute some points made by affirmative speaker.

iii.) state what affirmative must prove.

iv) state the position of your team on the question; show where you agree with affirmative.

v.) give main propositions in case.

b.) Discussion

i) present contentions and support.

c.) Conclusion

i) summarize argument and progress made.

2.) Second Negative Speech

a.) Introduction

i.) refute some argument by affirmative.

ii.) recall burden of proof.

iii.) summarize argument of colleague.

b.) Discussion

i.) state and support propositions.

c.) Conclusion

i.) summarize and show progress.

C. Refutation or Rebuttal

1.) Steps in effective refutation.

a.) State accurately and concisely the argument you propose to refute.

b.) State the importance of this argument and its bearing on your opponent's case.

c.) Refute the argument.

d.) Conclude by showing the effect on opponent's case.

2.) Methods

a.) Apply tests of evidence and reasoning to arguments of opponent's by showing:

i.) insufficient evidence.

ii.) doubtful sources.
iii.) drawing wrong conclusions.
iv.) incomplete or faulty analysis of the question.

**Modifications**

- Modify time for each speech.
- Only one debater per side. This requires more time between constructive speeches and rebuttals to allow debaters to organize their thoughts.

**Other Related Methodologies:** Disputation.

**References**


Archbold, P., & Hoeffer, B. (1981). Reframing the issue: A debate on third-party reimbursement. Nursing Outlook, 29 (7), 423-425.

Caffo, B. (1988). Philosophy debated: A teaching strategy. Nurse Educator, 13 (1), 29+.

Cooper, S. (1979). Methods of teaching-revisited, formal discussion: The debate. Journal of Continuing Education in Nursing, 10 (4), 58+.

Ewbank, H., & Auer, J. J. (1951). Discussion and debate: Tools for democracy. New York: Appleton Century Crofts.

Gesse, T., & Depsey, P. (1981). Debate as a teaching-learning strategy. Nursing Outlook, 29 (7), 421-423.

McBurney, O'Neill, & Mills. (1955). Argumentation and debate: Techniques of a free society. New York: MacMillan.

McIntosh, D., & Pettit, L. (1984). Research proposals and debate: A teaching strategy. Nursing & Health Care, 5 (6), 327-329.

Pender, N. (1967). The debate as a teaching and learning tool. Nursing Outlook, 15 (12), 42-43. (Junior students at the University of North Dakota participated in a debate about a public health issue. Preparation and learning outcomes are described.)

Wood, R. (1972). Strategic debate. Skokie, IL: National Textbook Co. (A basic text on debate. Contains descriptions of fundamentals of debate and strategies that might be used.)

# DEMONSTRATION

## Definition

*Demonstration* is the procedure of doing something in the presence of others either as a means of showing them how to do it themselves or in order to illustrate a principle. (Good)

## Purposes

- Teach psychomotor skills
- Convey information.
- Provide appreciation for approaches and processes.
- Define a problem in concrete terms.

## Responsibilities of the Teacher

- Plan practice demonstration to allow adequate time for unhurried presentation, questions, repeating segments if necessary.
- Prepare materials, equipment and physical environment.
- Prepare students.
- If students are demonstrating, obtain cooperation and permission.

## Concerns for Effective Learning

- Can all see and hear?
- Should chalkboard, outlines, and/or drawings be included?
- Pay particular attention to terms, parts and processes.
- Watch for obvious signs of confusion, disbelief, inattention.
- Talk to students, not to equipment or materials.
- Use good showmanship.
- Clarify concepts with slides, films, transparencies.
- Build up suspense by questioning.
- Concern for time limits, pacing.
- Review main steps during and/or at conclusion.
- Pass around some materials (e.g., very small parts, those which need to be felt).
- Students need to have time to try and/or apply learning.
- Is there an easier method (time and expense) -- film, filmstrip, videotape?
- May combine effectively with inquiry and discovery learning.

## Preparation

- Knowledge of purpose -- give the objectives for the demonstration.
- Plan for interest and attention (may include asking key questions).
- Knowledge of expectation for their participation.
  a. determining goal or purpose.
  b. participating during demonstration.
    1. note taking
    2. discussion

c. participating in demonstration or after completion.

**References**

Dale, E. (1969). Audio visual methods in teaching (3rd ed., pp. 271-293). New York: Dryden Press. (Basic information including use of tools to be used in demonstration, i.e., chalkboard.)

Good, C. V. (1959). Dictionary of education (2nd ed.). New York: McGraw-Hill.

Kilbourne, L. (1972). Can you teach a man to put on a coat without actually showing him how? Inservice Training and Education, 1 (1), 52-58.

Dave, R. H. (1971). In developing and writing performance objectives (pp. 20-21). Tucson, AZ: Educational Innovators Press. (Psychomotor variables of behavior in 5 levels, based on the concept of coordination.)

Gundmundsen, A. (1975). Teaching psychomotor skills. Journal of Nursing Education, 14 (1), 23-27.

Harrow, A. J. (1972). A taxonomy of the psychomotor domain. New York: David McKay Company. (A book on the psychomotor domain with taxonomy, entitled "Classification Levels of Psychomotor Domain.")

Moore, M. R. (1970). The perceptual-motor domain and a proposed taxonomy of perception. AV Communication Review, 18 (4), 379-411. (Proposes a perceptual taxonomy with the following categories: 1) sensation, 2) figure perception, 3) symbol perception, 4) perception of meaning, and 5) perceptive performance.)

Reilly, D. E. (1975). Behavior objectives in nursing: Evaluation of learner attainment (pp. 69-72). New York: Appleton, Century, Crofts. (A nurse author uses Dave's psychomotor levels.)

Robb, M. (1972). The dynamics of motor-skill acquisition. Englewood Cliffs, NJ: Prentice-Hall. (An approach to physical education skills based on Simpson's 7 phase taxonomy of psychomotor behaviors.)

Simmons, E. S. (1977). The effects of kinetic structure on knowledge about the performance of a psychomotor skill: Teaching students to use the compound microscope. Educational Horizons, 55 (3), 156-162. (The report of a study teaching high school students to use microscope.)

# DIARY

## Definition

*Diary* is a day to day recording by a student detailing selection of activities and relationships; such accounts usually revolve around: a) nature of the activity, b) purpose of the activity, c) outcome of activity, and d) student's feelings and attitudes about the activity. (Good)
*Personal Journal* is another form of diary. It may reflect thoughts on a specific topic area rather than day to day recording.

## Purposes

- Provide the learner with the opportunity to express reactions, thoughts, and feelings, and to receive feedback and assistance from the teacher.
- Provide the teacher with continuous, first hand data on which to base decisions for directing learning (determining the kinds and amount of assistance needed).
- Foster sensitivity in an "On-the-job" setting.
- Provide teacher with identification of satisfying and stressful clinical experiences.

---

**Advantages**

- Give evidence of how students are using concepts.
- Encourage systematic efforts to relate lecture content and reading assignments to clinical practice.
- Provide a form of written communication between student and teacher.
- Provide a teaching supplement to clinical teaching.
- Provide the teacher with examples and a realistic view.
- Individualize in area of sensitive and personal aspects of learning.
- Staff and agency attitudes, values, and ideas may be indicated.
- Contents of the diaries may be for personal use only or shared with group members in a variety of ways and for various purposes.

**Disadvantages**

- Trust is essential for open, frank sharing.
- Is a very private tool for the student to write and the teacher to read.
- The teacher may be tempted to push students to share.
- May be time consuming for students if diary is lengthy with frequent entries.
- Especially time consuming for teacher when many diaries are obtained.

---

## Points to Remember

- Relationship of the diary to the course objectives needs to be clear -- nature and purpose.
- A trust level must be built.
- Give specific instructions as to how much detail, how often to enter (daily, weekly, sample) over what time period and how the instructor will respond.

- Read, respond, and return promptly.
- The diary is not a substitute for clinical teaching.
- Obtain permission to use incident or ask student to share the incident.
- There is value in using over a time period, to see change in learners.
- Group members may determine how they will be used in class -- establishing ground rules.
- A personal diary, may be for the individual's use only and never submitted to the teacher.

**Other Related Methodologies:** Personal Journal.

**References**


Baumann, V. H. (1976). The professor and 100 students. Improving College and University Teaching, 24 (3), 145-146+. (Large lecture class adds diaries and reading reports.)

Burkhalter, P. K. (1975). Fostering staff sensitivity to the dying patient. Supervisor Nurse, 6 (4), 54-56. (A brief section suggesting the journal or diary.)

Crowley, D. M. (1965). Clinical diaries -- As part of the teaching-learning process. Journal of Nursing Education, 4 (4), 19-21. (Describes how the author used the diary.)

Good, C. V. (1973). Dictionary of education (3rd ed.). New York: McGraw-Hill.

Jackson, R. (1987). Approaching clinical teaching and evaluation through the written word: A humanistic approach. Journal of Nursing Education, 26 (9), 384-385.

Laughery, W. W., & Cromwell, R. E. (1970). Reflections of a student teacher. The Journal of Teacher Education, 21 (1), 34-43.

Rose, P. (1962). Using the student diary to identify stress-satisfaction. American Journal of Nursing, 62 (8), 94-96.

# DISCUSSION

**Definition**

*Discussion* is an activity characterized by adherence to a topic, question, or problem about which the participants sincerely wish to arrive at a decision or conclusion. (Good)

**Purpose**

- Use the resources of members of the group.
- Give students opportunities to formulate applications of principles.
- Get prompt feedback on how well objectives are being attained.
- Help students learn to think by giving them practice in thinking.
- Help students learn to evaluate the logic of and evidence for their own and others' positions.
- Help students become aware of and to formulate problems which necessitate information to be gained from readings or lectures.
- Gain acceptance for information or theories counter to folklore or previous beliefs of students.
- Develop motivation for further learning.

---

**Advantages**

- Provides opportunity for interchange of ideas and opinions based on varied experiences of group members.
- Stimulates interest in subject matter through direct involvement.
- Students may learn more and remember longer than with most other methods.
- Allows for individual freedom of expression.
- Gain feelings of acceptance and belonging.

**Disadvantages**

- Suitable ideally for a small group.
- Not as effective a method for some content -- i.e. instructions, procedural operations.
- May require a longer time to clarify and arrive at conclusions.
- May confuse some learners.
- Requires competent leadership.
- Leader (teacher) has less "control" of content.
- Not as useful presenting new information when student already is motivated to learn.

---

**Responsibilities of the Leader**

Prepare for leadership by:

a. Consider who the participants are, their backgrounds.
b. Study the topic, prepare questions if appropriate.

c. Introduce the topic, start the discussion.
d. Depending on "control" on the discussion, leader may wish to:
   1) pose questions.
   2) acknowledge contributions.
   3) encourage participation.
   4) refrain from indicating his biases.
   5) summarize occasionally.
   6) bring group back to topic or issue under discussion.
   7) assist in "handling" emotional reactions, arguments.

**The Instructor's Role**

The instructor's role will vary depending upon which of these or other functions the discussion is serving. The teacher as:

- v Expert
- v Authority
- v Socializing agent
- v Facilitator
- v Ego Ideal
- v Person (McKeachie, P. 38)

**Other Related Methodologies:** Panel, Seminar, Buzz Groups.

**References**


Cooper, R. M. (Ed.). (1958). The two ends of the log (pp. 32-33, 254-261). Minneapolis, MN: University of Minnesota Press. (Keith Taylor describes learning through discussion.)

French, S. (Ed.). (1954). Accent on teaching (pp. 23-56). New York: Harper and Brother. (Describes the thought process of students in discussion. Reports a study of student behaviors.)

Hill, W. F. (1962). Learning through discussion. Beverly Hills, CA: Sage Publications. (A basic guidebook for students and teachers who wish to use this method.)

Good, C. V. (1959). Dictionary of education (2nd ed.). New York: McGraw-Hill.

Leypoldt, M. M. (1967). 40 ways to teach in groups. Valley Forge, PA: Judson Press.

McKeachie, W. J. (1969). Teaching tips (6th ed., pp. 37-81). Lexington, MA: D.C. Health & Co. (A very complete discussion of the topic, including the research done.)

Parsons, J. (1976). A new approach to group learning. Journal of Continuing Education in Nursing, 7 (4), 5-9. (Using Roger's ideas in "Freedom to Learn," the author speaks to the teacher as the facilitator of learning and the students as a community of learners.)

Sanders, N. M. (1966). Classroom questions. New York: Harper & Row. (Relates the climate and learning in discussion to the kinds of questions posed.)

Stanford, G., & Stanford, B. (1969). Learning discussion skills through games. New York: Citation Press. (A sequence of games and techniques developed by two secondary school English teachers to help students develop discussion skills.)

Sullivan, P., & Beeler, J. (1979). Methods of teaching revisited: A format for discussion. Journal of Continuing Education in Nursing, 10(5), 15-17.

Carin, A., & Sund, R. (1971). Developing questioning techniques. Columbus, OH: Charles E. Merrill Publishing Co. (Using Bloom's domains, the authors suggest specific questioning techniques.)

Cooper, S. (1978). Methods of teaching-revisited, informal discussion. Journal of Continuing Education in Nursing, 9 (5), 14-16.

Rubin, F., et al. (1971). The seminar process -- An aid to learning. Nursing Outlook, 19 (1), 7. (A report of the use of the seminar process in one baccalaureate program.)

# DISPLAY

## Definition

*Display* (or exhibit) refers to a collection of related items displayed to aid learning. Display usually refers to flat, or two-dimensional materials; while exhibit connotes three-dimensional materials. Materials displayed may be reading materials, objects, produce, artifacts, products (learner made or manufactured), collections, instruments, and many others.

## Purposes

- Catch attention.
- Convey information quickly and simply.
- Convey concepts in more than one dimension to increase cognitive learning.
- Provide materials which are not generally available to learners.
- Inspire and stimulate individuals to think, change, and/or do something (ask questions, buy a product, visit, register, write, etc.).

---

**Advantages**

- Exposure to many people possible.
- Quickie way to promote ideas.
- Stimulates interest.
- Flexible and portable.
- Products and ideas of learners can be used.

**Disadvantages**

- Time consuming.
- May be expensive to organize and set up.
- May be disruptive to ongoing traffic and operations.
- Requires flexible space.

---

## Points to Remember

- Planning
  a. Relate plans to objectives or goals of the class or meeting.
  b. Begin planning well in advance. If several exhibits, have someone who is coordinator.
  c. Consider needs, interests, desires, and educational level of viewers.
  d. Select a theme to unify the exhibit.
  e. Determine best location, amount of space needed, lighting, etc.
  f. Sketch plans on paper to ensure unity and cohesion. If large booth type, build a scale model first and modify as necessary.
  g. Utilize learners (and their projects) in planning, making, and using the display whenever possible.
- Preparation of Materials
  a. Keep message short and simple with main idea stated clearly in minimum of words.

b. Select colors that go well together and are appropriate.
c. Blank space is often effective. Avoid an exhibit that is "too busy."
d. If using photographs, use only dull (matte) photos, not glossy ones.
e. All lettering should be easy to read and attractive.
    1) For attention, have some words or letters larger than others.
    2) Minimum letter height should be 1 inch for each 25 feet of viewing distance.
    3) Be sure all words are spelled correctly and letters correctly placed.
f. Add motion and sound as appropriate.
g. Label all items which might not be immediately recognizable.
h. Light exhibit adequately.
i. Take a picture of finished exhibit for own records.

➢ Promoting Exhibit

a. Encourage serious viewing of exhibit by setting aside time.
b. Might combine exhibit with a person to answer questions when necessary.
c. Dismantle before it becomes shopworn or overly familiar.

**Possible Criteria** -- if exhibit is to be judged

- Unit and cohesion.
- Attractive and neat.
- Appealing to the senses.
- Accurate information.
- Representative of theme.
- Location where exhibit is visible and unobtrusive to traffic.

**References**

Bergevin, P., Morris, D., & Smith, R. M. (1963). Adult education procedures (pp. 212-214). New York: Seabury Press. (A brief discussion of this educational teaching aid.)

Brown, C., & Pellion, T. (1984). CE in exhibit halls. Medical Meetings, 11, 34-35.

Cooper, S. (1981). Methods of teaching-revisited, displays and exhibits. Journal of Continuing Education in Nursing, 12, 35-37.

Dale, E. (1969). Audio-visual methods in teaching (3rd ed., pp. 580-581). New York: Dryden Press.

DeSantis, L., & Pett, D. (1981). Graphic thoughts. Development Communication Report, 3, 15.

Kinder, J. (1965). Audio-visual materials and techniques (3rd ed., pp. 162-164). New York: American Book Co. (Teachers use of display/exhibits is discussed.)

McCrudden, L. (1976). Health exhibit cuts a figure. Educational Horizons, 55 (1), 44-46.

# DISPUTATION

## Definition

*Disputation* is a method of verbal combat indulged in by many philosophers of ancient Athens. Sometimes a single reasoner alternately presents both sides of argument, but usually two or more disputants defend different points of view.

## Purposes

- Stimulates inquisitiveness.
- Teaches critical thinking and problem solving.
- Promotes inductive reasoning.
- Encourages learners to generalize.

---

**Advantages**

- Disputation is conducive to learning by discovery.
- It provides a change in teaching method from lecture.
- It is basically easy to use.
- It is useful in small or large groups (large groups may be subdivided).
- It requires learners to prepare arguments beforehand.

**Disadvantages**

- Learners may need orientation to the method.
- Time to prepare is needed -- the disputants can't come in "cold."

---

## Format

- Stimulus
  a. Students are given a statement to think about (e.g., "A patient with a new diagnosis of stroke should have the head of his bed elevated").
  b. All students choose (or are assigned to) a positive position, a negative position, or the role of moderator.
- Investigation
  a. Students are given two or three weeks to research the topic and amass evidence to support their position.
  b. Students also study the statement in depth to discover underlying principles, assumptions, generalities.
  c. Moderator prepares for both sides.

- Presentation
  a. One student each is selected to present positive and negative positions.
     1) Scientific support is expected.
     2) Empirical data are used cautiously.
     3) Solely observational or experienced evidence is discouraged.
  b. After presentation, moderator opens topic to discussion.
  c. Moderator summarizes the discussion and states a general conclusion or solution.
- Generalization of conclusion to apply to other situations.

**Responsibilities**

Teacher:
a. Present the topic in a yes-or-no manner.
b. Schedule topics and outline rules.
c. Clarify own role during the session.
d. Prepare and be knowledgeable about the topic.
e. During the disputation you may serve as resource person, build stimulant, but need not participate.

Learner:
a. Prepare position.
b. Bring necessary materials to disputation.

**Other Related Methodologies:** Mini Disputation, Debate.

**References**


Blauch, L. E. (1945). Teaching in colleges and universities (pp. 148-149). Indianapolis, IN: American Association of Dental Schools.

Veith, S. (1974). Disputation. Nursing Outlook, 22 (11), 699-701. (A nurse educator tells of her use of the method.)

# DRAMATIZED EXPERIENCES

## Definition

*Dramatized experiences* are instructional experiences using some form of play or acting, where students are the prime teaching tools.

## Purposes

- Provides opportunity to go, in thoughts and ideas, beyond the limits of the dimension of time.
- Assists learners to experience ideas and events they cannot confront directly in "true" form.
- Adds interest and zest to class work, a non-writing activity.
- Involves the creative and artistic talents of learners.
- Promotes unity and cooperation of learners through group work.
- Introduces content for discussion and exploration.

---

## Advantages

- Knowledge and experience are presented so that the audience is emotionally involved.
- Ideas may be placed in situations more readily identifiable with viewers' experiences.
- Abstract concepts and theories may be converted to real-life situations.
- Viewers are able to gain insight into other people's feelings and attitudes.
- Involvement of group members in the drama strengthens cohesiveness of the group.
- Plays are versatile and may be staged without elaborate script, scenery, or equipment.
- Dramatizations are suitable to groups of any age and size.
- Almost all individuals in a group can be worked into drama.
- Dramas provide a variety of experiences and responses; roles may be rotated among actors, helpers, and audience.

## Disadvantages

- Emotional power of drama can easily distort true facts and purpose, or slant them in a manner not intended or anticipated.
- Dramas cannot be used successfully with groups containing many inhibited or frightened persons.
- Overuse may lead to loss of novelty value.
- Formal dramatic productions (such as full-length plays) may require much work, time, cost, and equipment.
- Some learners may be uncomfortable with this type of activity.

---

## Performance Logistics

- The form of dramatized experience will determine the amount, kind, and complexity of equipment and assistance needed
- The teacher may need to work with the group to select a director. She may need to assist with other activities also.
- Group members may need to determine responsibilities of the director and other members.
- Stage area needs to be clearly seen, perhaps raised, and to have good lighting.
- The audience must be able to hear the performers' words. Actors need to rehearse with amplification if it is being used.
- It may be desirable to combine production with videotaping, audio taping, and/or photographs.

## Other Related Methodologies

Full-length play or formal dramatic production: One-, two-, or three-act play rehearsed and presented. Requires a director, cast of performers, and assistants.

Playlet: A short dramatic play, a small-scale production to treat a small problem or a small segment of a larger problem.

Dramatic skit: Use of dialogue and action to interpret situations and events rehearsed in advance and usually playing heavily on emotions. Short scenes.

Dialogue: Conversation with two or more persons.

Monologue (or characterization): One person dramatizes a specific personality.

Extemporaneous dramatization: Impromptu acting by preschool or early-school-age children.

Pageant: A story told by narrator and acted out by any number of persons on stage. A semiformal display involving drama, costumes, and music. Usually best for older students. May be elaborate and expensive. Usually requires a large number of persons.

Tableau: Usually a still picture, a grouping of persons and scenery. A narrator does all the speaking.

Pantomime: Actors express themselves with mute gestures, often accompanied by music. Useful for shy students. Doesn't require rehearsals, staging, or costuming. May be used in almost any classroom and many learning situations.

Role playing The assuming, either in imagination or overtly, on the part of another or others. (See guideline by that title).

Simulation games: Games where various aspects of drama play a part, such as role playing, dramatization, and extemporaneous play.

## Points to Remember

- Correlate drama with classroom objectives.
- Try to evoke emotions in the play that most of the viewers can sense themselves.
- For amateurs, staging should be simple, script flexible, and action as spontaneous as possible.
- Avoid exaggeration and sensationalism in serious matters.

- Enlist inhibited or bashful group members in drama by using them as stagehands, prompters, lighting experts,

- Carefully select, prepare, or modify the dramatic materials. It must be appropriate in content for both players and audience.
- Know the copyright laws relating to use and purchase of copies and payment of royalties.
- Tell the group how you will assist in preparation and production of play.
- The audience needs to be informed (via program or announcement) of:
  a. Background, principle players and casting.
  b. Whether or not they are to participate; if so, how and when?
- Take responsibility for discussion to follow. This may involve finding other discussion leaders. Discussion is a must!

**References**


Bauer, B. B. (1971). The educational play. Journal of Continuing Education in Nursing 2 (6), 46-48. (Reports on one of the "plays for living" the author used.)

Kalish, B. J. (1974). Summer theater: Another way to learn. Nursing Outlook, 22 (1), 31-34. (A faculty member in an associate degree program reports on the use of six one-act plays.)

Kinder, J. S. (1973). Using instructional media (pp. 165-170). New York: D. Van Nostrand, Co. (Basic material on several dramatic forms.)

Kidd, R. (1977, January). Popular theatre and development: A Botswana case study (PMB 0043). Gaborone, Botswana. (Used an annual folk festival to teach via drama, puppetry, music.)

Lewis, F. M. (1977). A time to live and a time to die: An instructional drama. Nursing Outlook, 25 (12), 762-765. (The author describes the use of a 16-minute original play to teach about death and care of the dying patient.)

Morgan, B., Holmes, G. E., & Bundy, C. E. (1976). Methods in adult education (3rd Ed). Danville, IL: Interstate Printers & Publishers. (A useful source of information about drama and adult learners.)

# FABLE

**Definition**

*Fable* is a brief story or tale feigned or invented to embody a moral; and introducing persons, animals, or sometimes even inanimate things as rational speakers and actors.

**Purposes**

- For diversion only in early history.
- Taught cultural and moral sense.
- Taught practical aspects of life.
- Often adds humor.

---

**Advantages**

- An old method of teaching which can always be contemporary.
- Short, quickly read or told.
- Appeals to the imagination.
- Appropriate non-literate form of learning; the oral tradition in teaching.
- Versatile and practical.
- Requires no equipment or advance preparation to those able to ad lib.
- May be combined with audiovisuals if appropriate.

**Disadvantages**

- Is an inductive method of teaching.
- May be difficult to locate appropriate prepared fables.
- Those who intend to prepare their own need to be familiar with both the structure of fables and the cultural context of their use.

---

**Points to Remember**

- Sources include ancient (Greek, Jewish, Buddhist, Hindu) and modern (England, Russian, France, US) fables.
- Teachers may locate fables written specifically for education, health, and other areas.

**Other Related Methodologies:** Folk Tales, Allegory, Parable, Storytelling, Fairy Tales.

**References**

Mager, R. (1962). Preparing instructional objectives. Palo Alto, CA: Fearon Pub. (A Sea Horse fable in the preface is an example of an educational fable.)

Nowlin, C. (1929). The story teller and his pack (pp. 187-240). Springfield, MS: Milton Bradley Co. (An excellent source of information about the history and use of fables.)

Yolen, J. (1986). Favorite Folk tales from Around the World. NY: Pantheon Books.

# FAIRY TALES

**Definition**

*Fairy Tales* are narratives in which the supernatural is an essential part. (Sometimes used loosely to include folk tales, fables, myths and legends).

**Purposes**

- In ancient times:
  a) explain mysterious phenomena
  b) entertain, escape monotony, give pleasure, amuse
- In later times:
  a) direct to discover identity
  b) internalize processes that are external and thus make them comprehensible
  c) teach practical aspects of life

---

**Advantages**

- Traditional, one of the oldest forms of literature.
- Universal, (not all are written down).
- Requires imagination and stirs emotions.
- Uses various ethnic/cultural groups as examples (i.e., Native American).
- Few plot elements or formula necessary.

**Disadvantages**

- May want to know where they come from and the relationship to ancient man's thinking.
- Need to evaluate those used (some have racial biases, cruelty).
- Since they develop attitudes and suggest improving behavior, may have both positive and negative valence attached to them.

---

**Components of a Typical Fairy Tale**

- Preliminary situation
- Initial episode
- Steps in rising action
- Climax
- Falling action
- Conclusion

**Characteristics**

- Optimistic, happy ending
- Variously classified
- Leave the decisions up to the listener

**Other Related Methodologies:** Myths, Modern Animal Tales, Folk Tales, Legends, Fables

**References**

Bettelheim, B. (1977). The uses of enchantment, the meaning and importance of fairy tales. New York: Vantage Books.

Fisher, L., & Reichenbach, M. (1987/1988). From Tinkerbell to Rogers. (How a fairy tale facilitated an understanding of Roger's Theory of Unitary Being). Nursing Forum, 13 (1), 1-9.

Heinrich, K., & Killeen, M. (1993). The gentle art of nurturing yourself. American Journal of Nursing, 10, 41-43.

Lomuto, J. (1975). Fairy tales can come true. Training and Development Journal, 29 (9), 46-47. (A fairy tale about managers and "the organization.")

Nowlin, C. (1929). The story teller and his pack (p. 293). Springfield, MA: Milton Bradley Co.

Olendzki, M. (1973). Cautionary tales. Wakefield, MA: Contemporary Pub., Inc. (Humorous tales related to health care. Many appeared in other journals. However, some authors do not consider cautionary tales as fairy tales.)

Wright, D. (1993). "The princess and the chemo spill" -- A policy magically turned into a fairy tale. Journal of Continuing Education in Nursing, 24, 27-38.

Yolen, J. (1986). Favorite Folktales from Around the World. NY: Pantheon Books.

# FIELD NOTES

## Definition

*Field Notes* is an expanded account of the client interview, which contains the data to be used for analysis.

## Procedure

- Data should include:
  a. An accurate account of the client's conversation, expressions of his/her experience, and nonverbal communication.
  b. The observer's impressions of the informant and the observed responses of others to the informant.
  c. The observer's analysis and interpretation of the data, and hypotheses formulated to be tested in future interviews.
  d. Client impressions need not go on after first couple of weeks.
- Process to be followed:
  a. Please leave wide margins to permit room for instructor comments. Need not be typed -- write legibly.
  b. Submit a copy of the field notes weekly to the instructor (at least every other week).
  c. Instructor will return within a week.
  d. Content may be discussed in conferences (held every other week, generally the week after submission of notes.).

## References


Field (1983). An Ethnography: four public health nurses perspectives of nursing. Journal of Advanced Nursing. 8, 3-12.

Leininger (1985). Ethnography and ethnonursing: models and modes of qualitative data analysis, pp. 33-71. (in Leininger, M. (ed.), Qualitative research methods in nursing 1985. New York: Grune and Stratton).

Robertson and Boyle (1984). Ethnography: contribution to nursing research, Journal of Advanced Nursing, 9, 43-49.

Spradley, J. (1979). The ethnographic interview. New York: Holt, Reinhart, & Winston.

# FIELD TRIP

## Definition

*Field Trip* is an investigation away from the classroom; the transportation of learners to places where the materials of instruction may be observed and studied directly in their functional setting. (Good). Synonymous with study tour.

## Purposes

- Observe the actual process.
- Gather information by observing real source materials, concrete evidence, situations, or individuals.
- Visit places whose activities demonstrate the attitudes and values you wish to emphasize.
- Provide access to new ideas and methods that have developed but are not available in print or other media.

---

## Advantages

- Provides a direct observation experience.
- Demonstrates "real life."
- Stimulates interest.
- Clarifies aspects which may be difficult to comprehend or believe.
- Increases understanding of specifics and broadens general background knowledge.
- Stimulates new ideas, further study, and/or more effective performance.
- Study objects, materials, processes or people within their natural environment.

## Disadvantages

- Is time consuming.
- May be costly, especially if careful preparation is not made.
- May distract attention from main objectives (other aspects may catch attention).
- May be disruptive to ongoing operations, inconvenience or disturb those being observed.
- May result in poor public relations.

---

## Criteria for Site Selection

- Suitable for the objectives and content.
- Can be completed in the allotted time.
- Valuable enough to justify the time of the class and teacher.
- Suitable to the interest and level of the learner.
- Either a representative location with general applications or a unique setting.

## Planning the Trip

Preliminary Planning

a. Make preliminary contacts (including an advance tour for the teacher if necessary) well in advance.
b. Arrange for details of scheduling, number to be accommodated, transportation, finances, permissions.
c. Provide the tour guide with the objectives of the tour and information about the learners.

Prepare the Group

a. Discuss the objectives of the trip.
b. When necessary, give preliminary lectures, instructions, and/or assignments (readings).
c. Give specific instructions on what to observe, what specific object is or activities to note.
d. Provide guide sheets if appropriate.
e. Include a discussion with the tour guide during the tour, if appropriate.

Follow-up Activities

a. As soon as possible, after the tour, follow up with a discussion and evaluative session (may include a report or quiz).
b. Identify new interests, unplanned or unexpected learners, and groups.
c. Record evaluation in resource file.
d. Write appropriate thank-you notes to individuals and agencies.

## References


Brown, J. W., et al. (1959). A-V instruction, materials and methods (pp. 362-368). New York: McGraw-Hill.

Dale, E. (1969). Audio-visual methods in teaching (3rd ed., pp. 296-321). New York: Dryden Press.

Good, C. (1959). Dictionary of education (2nd ed.). New York: McGraw-Hill.

Peoples, E., Jr. (1969). The bus lecture technique for teaching about life in the city. Journal of Nursing Education, 7, 15-20.

Schweer, J., & Gebbie, K. (1976). Creative teaching in clinical nursing (3rd ed., pp. 133-135). St. Louis: C.V. Mosby.

Wolf, L. (1948). The field trip. American Journal of Nursing, 48, 654.

# FLEXI-FLANS

## Definition

*Flexi-flans and maxi-flans* are cardboard actors which may depict a changing scene and/or tell a story. Flexi-flans are small figures (5-6 inches) and maxi-flans are large (20-24 inches). They are also known as jointed cardboard figures, or actionettes, and usually used on the flannel board.

## Purposes

- Activate stationary figures to allow depiction of a change in scenery.
- Express ideas thereby enhancing and facilitating the discussion of needs and problems.
- Activate flannel graph figures.

---

**Advantages**

- Involve learners in action of the figure and in discussion.
- Easily make culture and region specific.
- Easily portable (12-16 cm, or 50-60 cm).
- Reusable.

**Disadvantages**

- Preparation of original figures takes time.

---

## Points to Remember

- Visual means to express ideas by change of expression or action.
- Facilitate and enhance discussion.
- Obtain learners' opinions and solutions to resolve conflict.
- Flexi-flans used with flannel board, maxi-flans usually are not.
- Present different views of local customs and beliefs to encourage examination of influence on health.
- It is possible to make a good drawing from a paper doll model because the doll gives you correct proportions of human figure.

## Materials Needed

- Stiff paper cardboard for maxi-flans, and poster board, heavy construction, or blotter paper for flexi-flans.
- Pencils, pens, paints, etc.
- Scissors, shoe eyelets, metal fasteners, string or tread.
- Flannel or sandpaper for backing.
- Figures (people, common community objects, houses, trees, etc.)
- Flannel Board (large size if maxi-flans)

**Procedure**

- Write story.
- Prepare figures ahead of time.
  a. Prepare drawings -- color or paint.
  b. Paste on heavy paper.
  c. Cut out.
  d. Sandpaper or flannel on back.
- Introduce story.
- Students choose figures and put on flannel board depicting a problem or need.
- Discuss, have others move them, resolve conflict, discuss further.

**Other Related Methodologies:** Flannel Board.

**References**


Barclay, E. (1984). Easy to make teaching aids. Nutrition Education Series, #10. Paris: UNESCO, (pp. 18-24). Includes patterns and instructions.

Crone, C., & Hunter, C. (1980). From the field. Tested participatory activities for trainers New York: World Education.

Scrinivasan, L. (1982). Bridging the gap: A participatory approach to health and nutrition education. Washington, DC: Save the Children Federation, USA.

Unknown. (n.d.) Drawing form a paper doll model. In Action, 19, 4-6.

Unknown. (1994, June). Pictures with model figures. Footsteps, 19. 8-9.

Werner, D., & Bower, B. (1982). Helping health workers learn. Palo Alto, CA: Hesperian Foundation.

# FILING AND STORING

## Definition

*Filing* is a system used to arrange and store materials (such as papers, booklets, records, instructions and audiovisual materials) -- may be alphabetical, numeric, geographic, subject, date or some other order. (Implies collecting, organizing, and storing.)

## Purposes

- Provide ready and easy access to materials.
- Utilize storage space efficiently.

---

**Advantages**

- Facilitates availability, and therefore, utilization of materials.
- Conserves time.
- Saves duplication.
- A well functioning system keeps storage problems at a minimum.
- Provides best care for materials -- preserves and protects.
- Inexpensive systems and undesirable space may be used.
- Enhances use of materials by more than one individual.

**Disadvantages**

- Collectors may keep more materials and not discard.
- Collecting indiscriminately often occurs -- thus lessening the effectiveness of the filing system.
- Filing requires space.
- Storing requires space.
- Files and storage closets may be expensive.

---

## Suggestion for Use

- There are many filing plans, the important thing is to find one which fits the individual and the materials to be filed.
- Those who have a variety of materials may need more than one filing/storing system.
- Filing must be accompanied by pruning, preferably on a specific schedule.
- Those fortunate enough to have secretarial help with filing need an explainable system.
- As a general rule, keep pacesetting articles, definitive articles, difficult to obtain items, and items by experts.
- Document fully all materials to avoid waste of time in giving proper credit. (Full title, author, pages, source, cost, key factors to be remembered).

**Other Related Methodologies:** Filing System, Collections, Collecting, Storage.

**References**


Beatty, L. F. (1978, February). An easy-to-make instructional materials file. Audio-visual instruction, 23 (2), 30+.

Dorff, P. (1982). File! Don't pile! A personal filing system. Minneapolis: Willowtree Press, Inc. (Highly recommended). (A local librarian, lecturer, and consultant writes material she has used in workshops on the topic of the filing system.)

Gustafson, M. (1988). File it, Don't pile it!! Journal of Continuing Education in Nursing 19 (5), 233-234.

Hoyt, J.S., Jr. (1977). Personal time management and effective administration (6th ed.). Minneapolis, MN: University of Minnesota, Ag. Extension Services. (Author suggests his elaborate filing system.)

Humphrey, N.D. (1979, February). The biological basis of collecting. Human Nature, 2 (2), 44-47. (Interesting article with special reference to usual collectors -- such as stamps, coins.)

McGinn, H.F. (1975, June). A/V materials -- where should they be kept? Nursing Outlook, 23 (6), 38-39.

Narrow, B.W. (1979). Patient teaching in nursing practice, a patient and family centered approach (pp. 163-165). New York: Wiley. (A brief section on "Your Personal AV file" with suggestions on how to do it.)

# FILMS

## Definition

*Films* are consecutive pictures or photographs of objects in motion projected on a screen so rapidly as to give the illusion that the objects are moving as they did in the original scenes. May make use of sound as well as visual images. Synonymous with movie, motion pictures, films, "flicks".

## Purposes

- Bring the world to the classroom.
- Provide a common stimulus for all students.
- Provide for continuity and time lapse.
- Provide many specific examples.
- Develop moods and empathy.
- Demonstrate methods or skills.
- Reinforce and extend previous learning.
- Provide an economic, quick orientation.
- Provide a review or summary.
- Evaluate achievement of particular objectives.

---

**Advantages**

- Time saving; movies can present an edited version of reality and also eliminate travel to an actual setting.
- Heighten reality by eliminating distractions and by pointing out relationships that may otherwise be overlooked.
- Can achieve identification and involvement of the viewer with the situation presented.
- Can bring the distant past and the present into the classroom.
- Builds a common denominator of experience.
- Compels attention.
- Offers a satisfying aesthetic experience.

**Disadvantages**

- Expense of renting or buying the movie, and equipment.
- All information presented may not be consistent with desired subject.
- May present more material than learners can handle in a very short time.
- Mechanical difficulties may occur.
- The influence of a movie is specific, not general.
- Previewing requires time and may involve expense.

---

**Suggestions for Use**

- Essential to preview a movie before using it. Consider:
  a. Is it up to date?
  b. Is it accurate?
  c. Is it directed to the level of the learners?
  d. Is all or part of the content appropriate?
  e. Does it meet the objectives?
  f. How long is it?
  g. How much does it cost? (Rent or buy?)
  h. Can the cost be justified?
- May wish to prepare a printed study guide for use before and after viewing.
- Prepare the room and equipment for showing to be sure everything is in working order.
- Prepare learners for the movie.
  a. Why? -- relates it to the objectives.
  b. What? -- research indicates that learning increases when the viewers are told explicit points for which they are to watch.
  c. Define terminology which may be unfamiliar to viewers.
  d. Discourage note taking. McKeachie (1969) reports that research by Ash and Carlton indicates that note taking during a movie is not effective (p. 111).
  e. Indicate what follow-up activities will take place -- discussion, testing, etc.
- Remain in the room no matter how often have seen the movie -- absence may indicate disinterest.

**Modification**

- Dale (1969) states that research supports using movies in combination with other instructional materials for better learning (p. 412).

  Examples:
  a. Modified role play -- learners assigned to identify with particular characters in the movie.
  b. Show part of a movie. Have students complete the story as an exercise in creativity.
  c. Show the beginning of a movie. Have students use problem solving to come up with a diagnosis and solution. Then show the end of the movie to indicate what actually happened.
  d. Use only one segment of a movie for a particular purpose -- e.g., introduction to a class, illustrate a particular concept, etc.
- Repeating a film increases learning for less able learners.

**Sources of Movies**

- Professional Education Journals, e.g., American Journal of Nursing, Nursing Outlook.
- American Journal of Nursing Co., Education Services Division.
- State Department of Health Film Library.
- US Department of Health, Education and Welfare, International Film Bureau.

- University of Minnesota, Audiovisual Library Service.
- Drug companies.
- National Medical Audiovisual Center, National Library of Medicine, Atlanta, Georgia.
- Commercial film companies.
- TV stations or sponsors of particular programs.
- Card file of movies used. Helpful to keep on record the following information:
  a. Exact title.
  b. Source.
  c. Topic.
     1) short description of content.
     2) subject matter areas in which film could be used.
  d. Level of learner for whom it's most suited.
  e. Length.
  f. Cost.
  g. Producer and production date.
  h. Strong points.
  i. Weak points.
  j. Overall evaluation.

**References**


Arwady, J. (1980). The oral introduction to the instructional film: A closer look. Educational Technology, 20, 18-22.

Beck, L. (1966). Use of films and television for creative teaching. In C. Taylor & F. Williams (Eds.), Instructional media and creativity (Chapter 8). New York: John Wiley & Sons. (This article offers several specific examples of how films were used creatively at various levels of education. Explicit comments and reactions are helpful.)

Brown, J., et al. (1959). A-V instructional materials and methods (pp. 157-182). New York: McGraw-Hill. (This resource book offers quite a thorough description of the use of films for teaching.)

Dale, E. (1969). Audiovisual methods in teaching (3rd ed.). New York: The Dryden Press, Holt, Rinehart, & Winston.

del Bueno, D. (1976). No more Wednesday matinees. Nursing Outlook, 24 (6), 359-361. (Describes the typical in-service program of showing a film as entertainment, not staff development. Includes alternatives.)

Frey, M. (1969). Basic steps in film making. Nursing Outlook, 17 (5), 50-60. (If you choose to make your own film, this article offers tips on how to go about it.)

Kerpelman, L. (1975). Films in nursing education. Nursing Outlook, 23, 35-37. (Reports a survey of nurses who used the National Medical Audiovisual Center's film loan service. Reports types of programs using films and the effects of using films.)

Kubo, W., et al. (1971). A creative examination. Nursing Outlook, 19 (8), 524-526. (This article describes the evaluation of students' clinical performances through the use of the film, "The Special Universe of Walter Krolik" as a situational test.)

McKeachie, W. (1969). Teaching tips: A guidebook for the beginning college teacher (pp. 109-112). Lexington, MA: D.C. Health & Co. (Another general resource on films, not as complete as Brown. Incorporates research findings.)

Schweer, J., & Gebbie, K. (1976). Creating teaching in clinical nursing (3rd ed., pp. 140-142). St. Louis: C.V. Mosby Co.

# FILMSTRIP

**Definition**

*Filmstrip* is a series of slides joined together on one strip of film. Usually accompanied by a sound track on either cassette or record, or by a script.

**Purposes**

- Shows something that has happened.
- Develops and heightens attention.
- Encourages student participation.

---

**Advantages**

- A filmstrip is less expensive than a movie.
- Equipment is lightweight and portable.
- Showing is adapted to fit a particular setting by taking as much time as needed to study a process or procedure. Filmstrip may be stopped for discussion.
- Teacher and students may make their own filmstrip.
- Filmstrip projectors are simple to operate.
- Filmstrips are inexpensive to make, and numerous ones are available for purchase.
- Filmstrips may be combined with audio.
- They can be used for individual study or group viewing.
- They don't require much storage space.

**Disadvantages**

- Filmstrips cannot portray motion, just suggest it.
- Time is required to preview and/or prepare.
- A special projector is required. Some are combined with a slide projector.
- Tape and record audio accompaniments restrict use of filmstrips by controlling speed, giving the teacher less chance to clarify or extend ideas.
- Filmstrips may be damaged if not properly cared for and stored.
- Lack of synchronization with audio is at least temporarily confusing.
- The bell signal to advance may become annoying.

---

**Suggestions for Use**

- Read operating instructions carefully.
- Preview.
- Read guide that accompanies filmstrip, and script if available.
- Introduce, mention specific things to watch for, and raise questions.

- Stop and make comments if continuity will not be disturbed.
- Discuss filmstrip after viewing.
- Use creatively: Do not use entire filmstrip if not necessary.
- If you make your own, seek instructions available in audiovisual texts.
    a. Carefully organize pictures, vocabulary, and relationship between visual and verbal communication.
    b. You may make a filmstrip of anything drawn, written, typewritten, printed, or photographed.

**References**

Dale, E. (1976). Audiovisual methods in teaching (3rd ed., pp. 456-457). New York: Dryden Press, Holt, Rinehart & Winston.

Kinder, J. (1973). Using instructional media (pp. 69-71). New York: D. Van Nostrand.

Schweer, J. (1972). Creative teaching in clinical nursing (2nd ed., pp. 191-192). St. Louis: C.V. Mosby.

# FLANNEL BOARD

## Definition

*Flannel Board* is a portable, flat, board like object covered with long-fibered or napped cloth such as flannel, felt, or suede, to which appropriately backed items will adhere. Synonymous with flannel graph, felt board.

## Purposes

- Add visual aspect to a sequenced oral presentation.
- Build concepts step by step or by manipulation of the symbols.
- Teach a technical skill by having learners manipulate the symbols.
- Present symbolic clarification of ideas as an adjunct to other media, such as television.
- Illustrate a story as it is being told.
- Mount or display diagrams and charts.

---

## Advantages

- A flannel board permits two techniques for delivering a message: words (sound) and symbols or pictures (sight).
- It is appealing to any age group, particularly because audience watches steps in procedure or presentation.
- Any message told as a story can be transferred to flannel board.
- It challenges teacher to develop symbols to portray abstractions.
- Materials (and equipment) may be packed and transported easily.
- Chronological development of ideas promotes ease in note-taking.
- Flannel boards are inexpensive and may be homemade.
- Flannel board permits creativity and use of colors for specific purposes.
- Board may be combined with other media, such as music or a recorded story.

## Disadvantages

- A flannel board requires considerable ingenuity and imagination to construct effective and varied materials.
- Although tool is simple, teacher needs to be well organized and to practice.
- Convenience of use might tend to deter teacher from other, more effective methods and techniques.
- Presentation is limited -- a new idea involves a lapse of time before the new material can be made and added.
- Telling a complete story often takes either too much board space or small designs and materials, some of which cannot be seen well.
- Considerable time and cost may be involved in making material and equipment.

---

## Suggestions for Making Visuals

- Begin by developing an idea and then translating it into the flannel medium.
- Appropriate visuals and symbols may be drawn, found, or purchased ready-made (such as the Eli Lilly punch-out visuals of food exchanges for teaching diabetic patients).
- Find out whether the visual is copyright-free; if not, make appropriate arrangements for use.
- Sources might be clip-art source books used for journals or newspaper advertisements.
- Follow rules for use of other graphics for clarity, simplicity, and color contrasts.
- A file for pictures will save preparation time.
- Be concerned with the background -- generally use a dark, solid color.

## Suggestions for Making Boards

- The figures are more important than the equipment, but well-made equipment is easier and more enjoyable to use.
- School-supply stores sell a variety of boards at different prices.
- A standard-size board is 24 by 36 inches.
- Homemade boards may be made of various lightweight materials, such as beaver board, Celotex, Masonite, Bristol board, wallboard, or heavy cardboard.
- Boards can be covered with outing flannel, felt, suede cloth, or Vell-O, fastened securely to backing with staple guns, brads, glue, binding tape, or thumbtacks.
- Easels may be floor or table models, made of wood or metal. Ready-made ones are sold in many craft shops.
- Some audiovisual books have instructions for making easels.

## Suggestions for Using Visuals

- Use the flannel board when opportunity for follow-up is limited.
- Consider its use when message deals with abstract quantities and when it is hoped that change of attitudes and practices will eventually occur.
- Use as a supplement to what might otherwise be a rather boring lecture.
- Use to present major concepts in a process and/or to summarize material already covered.
- Be sure board is firmly fixed in well-lighted, clearly visible area with ample room to apply visual items.
- Each item should be numbered in order of use, ready for instant pickup and application at time it is discussed. Delays and interruptions of content to offer apologies for oversights should be avoided.
- Simplicity is the key to effective presentation.
- If board is placed at a slight angle, backgrounds and figures will adhere more readily.
- Stand to the side as you use the board; be sure everyone can see it and that height is right.
- Use rubber cement in applying flannel or other backing material to visual.
- An easel for a flip chart may double for the flannel board easel.

**Suggestions for Using Variety**

- A wide variety of materials will adhere, some of which are three-dimensional: yarn, pipe cleaners, foam rubber, sponges, embroidery floss, velvet, suede, sandpaper, felt, Styrofoam.
- Combine board with sound effects, musical background, or other media.
- Inexpensive small boards may be made for use with small groups and held in the teacher's lap. They can be made from grocery cartons, or use a flannel story apron or hinged cigar box.
- Some groups may wish to use the board on the floor without an easel.

**Other Related Methodologies:** Hook and Loop (Velcro) board.

**References**

Gdansk, L., & Hamamoto, P. (1977). The joys of flannel. Audiovisual Instruction, 22 (6), 42-43. (Suggests use of the flannel board with adults.)

Kinder, J. (1973). Using instructional media. New York: D. Van Nostrand, Co. (Ideas for use with all age groups.)

Morgan, B., Holmes, G., & Bundy, C. (1976). Methods in adult education (3rd ed., pp. 201-204). Danville, IL: Interstate Printers and Publishers. (Lists advantages and disadvantages of the flannel board.)

Schweer, J., & Gebbie, K. (1976). Creative teaching in clinical nursing (3rd ed., pp. 136-137). St. Louis, MO: C. V. Mosby. (Suggests ways to use the flannel board in clinical teaching.)

Size more, H. (1976). Teaching with flannel graph. Cincinnati, OH: Standard Publishing. (Suggestions for homemade boards and materials.)

# FLASH CARD

## Definition

*Flash Card* is a small card of stiff cardboard having on it written or printed letters, words, phrases, numerals, or combinations; used as an aid to learning by holding each card up for the class to see for a brief interval.

## Purposes

- As a tool for "drill" when content is to be memorized.
- Briefly illustrates main points in a lecture.

---

## Advantages

- Cards are simple and inexpensive to prepare.
- They are easy to handle.
- Both teachers and students can make them.
- They are useful for individual or group education.
- Learners may assist each other.
- Cards can be attractive and interesting.
- They may be used repeatedly and transported easily.
- Some materials are available for purchase.
- Cards may help slow or handicapped learners.
- Flash cards permit self-pacing and repeated use.

## Disadvantages

- Cards are useful primarily for younger learners.
- They can be distracting if there is too much detail.

---

## Suggestions for Use

- When teacher makes flash card:
  a. Make large enough for group use.
  b. Use sturdy tagboard or cardboard.
  c. Use bright colors, simple pictures and sketches.
  d. Be sure words are spelled correctly.
  e. Keep simple -- one word or short phrase.
- When to use:
  a. In teaching, reviewing, evaluating.
  b. By individuals outside class.
- May wish to use magnetic photo album for a flash card story.

**References**


Kinder, J. (1973). Using instructional media (pp. 65-67). New York: D. Van Nostrand.

Staton, T. (1960). How to instruct successfully. In Modern Teaching Methods (pp. 175-176). New York: McGraw-Hill.

Zaremba, D. (1970). Use flash cards to teach basic principles. Business Education Forum, 25 (3), 9-11.

# FLIP CHART

## Definition

*Flip Chart* is a series of bound-together sheets of paper or poster board which can be flipped over, one at a time, to show a series of thoughts, pictures, outline points, questions, cartoons, symbols or almost anything that helps teach.

## Purposes

- Permits demonstration of sequence or series.
- Allows for use of permanently mounting pictures, charts, poems and diagrams.
- For easy handling and transport of a series of flat pictures.
- A blank flip chart may be a good incentive in a brainstorming session.

---

**Advantages**

- A useful teaching tool that is portable, economical and versatile.
- A substitute for chalkboard.
- Can be prepared ahead of time and transported.
- Provides for permanence and repeated use.
- Useful with small audience.
- Conveys feeling of spontaneity when idea is listed immediately after contributed.

**Disadvantages**

- Not useful with large audiences.

---

## Responsibilities of the Teacher

- Print and use pictures or symbols that are large enough to be easily seen.
- Add bright colors to charts and symbols through use of crayons, colored felt pens, pasted-on colored paper, water colors or tempera.
- For a three-dimensional effect, scotch tape objects on the chart.
- For a problem-solving session, use stick figures or cartoon faces.
- In addition to displaying simple time charts, use fold-out sheets.
- Learners may make their own flip charts to review material or to pictorially present their own group or individual ideas.
- It may be both convenient and necessary to provide for an easel or stand (the cardboard cover may serve as an easel).

## Sources for Purchasing or Making

- Artist's large sketch pad at art supply store -- spiral bound and large enough for use with groups; usually of good, durable quality paper.

- Make your own from sheets of wrapping paper or newsprint clipped to an easel or bound to a piece of cardboard with binder rings.
- Use felt-tip pens, crayons, heavy pencil or tempera paint.

**References**

Lange, C. (1976). Developing low-cost teaching materials. (The Media Center). Nursing Outlook, 24 (10), 614.

Van Hoozer, H. (1982). Visual communication. Basic guidelines. Iowa City, IA: University of Iowa.

# FLOW CHART

## Definition

*Flow Chart* is a graphic media designed to visualize relationships of key facts and ideas as well as steps in a process or sequence. Synonymous with organizational chart

## Purpose

- Show sequence and relationship.
- Show steps in a process.
- Illustrate functional and administrative relationships.
- Show levels of authority, priority, and/or cause.

---

**Advantages**

- Show how parts are organized into a whole or steps of operations.
- Show responsibility or functional relationships.
- Show sequences (in time) or processes by combining boxes or drawings with lines or captions.

**Disadvantages**

- When too complicated or elaborate, may confuse.

---

## Points to Remember

- Avoid complicated drawings that will confuse.
- Keep it simple by using one idea.
- It is better to break a complicated chart into two or more simple ones.
- Do not try to include too much data.
- Use squares, rectangles, triangles and other symbols for each component.
- Compare like units to avoid confusion.

**Other Related Methodologies:** Chart, Algorithm, Decision Making Tree, Fishbone Diagram.

## References

Kinder, J. (1973). Using instructional media. New York: Van Nostrand.

Van Hoozer, H. (1982). Visual communications basic guidelines. Iowa City, IA: University of Iowa, College of Nursing.

Lane, G., Cronin, K., & Pierce, A. (1983). Flow charts: Clinical decision making in nursing. Philadelphia: Lippincott.

# FOLK TALE

**Definition**

*Folk Tale* is a primitive tale and form of primitive literature, often including myths, folk tales, and fairy tales. (Similar terms -- folk lore, folk literature).

**Purposes**

- Explain theories and beliefs, mostly animistic spirits.
- Pass down traditions and values.

---

**Advantages**

- Early, traditional form.
- Folk literature is the key to the working of the "primitive" mind.

**Disadvantages**

- Very similar to other forms of primitive literature, thus difficult to get a specific discussion of this form.
- Difficult to find examples and components of a typical folk tale.

---

**References**


Burris, N. A. (1985). Third-graders write folk tales. Educational Horizons, 64 (1), 32-35.

Janssen, A. T. (1981). International stories. Englewood Cliffs, NJ: Prentice Hall (A conversation-reader to improve your English, contains fables, folk tales, and folk stories.)

Johnson, G. (1949). How the donkeys came to Haiti and other tales. New York: Devin-Adair.

Nowlin, C. H. (1929). The story teller and his pack (pp. 164-183). Springfield, MA: Milton Bradley Co. (Example: Courlander, Harold. Uncle Bouqui of Haiti. Morrow).

Yolen, J. (1986). Favorite Folktales from Around the World. NY: Pantheon Books.

# GAMING

## Definition

*Game, simulation* is a specially designed activity providing opportunities to practice certain components of life itself by providing a set of players, a set of allowable actions, a segment of time, and a framework within which the action takes place; this leads students to active assimilation of information in order to carry out action toward relevant goals.

## Purposes

- Presents learning experiences specifically designed to represent actual problems.
- Teaches a process and gives experience in decision-making; emphasis on affective domain.
- Motivates students in study of historical or contemporary problems.
- Applies concepts and principles.
- Changes attitudes.
- Provides experiential learning -- learners experience anxiety, doubt, insecurity, etc.

---

## Advantages

- Gaming provides learner with essential aspects of a real situation without the hazards, costs, or time limitations.
- Games may be made by the teacher or commercially purchased.
- Many are inexpensive and reusable.
- Games challenge students of varying abilities.
- Games are versatile -- there are various types and ways to use them.
- They provide a relatively safe but standardized learning environment.
- Teacher can use games in a variety of ways.
- Games can be a refreshing change of pace.

## Disadvantages

- A game may be seen as an amusement only and not for educational purposes.
- Limited research exists on this methods value.
- Some games require certain furniture, large room, or special equipment.
- Some games may be costly, especially if large numbers need to be purchased.
- Games can be time-consuming for the teacher to evaluate, prepare, and/or carry out.
- Some teachers must overcome prejudices against games (they are a gimmick, too complicated, too noisy).
- Teachers may not recognize the full creative potential of gaming.

---

**Types of Games:** Card, Board, Floor.

**Points to Remember**

- Selection (or preparation) (See article by Ball for further suggestions).
  a. Rules should be clear and concise.
  b. Sufficient examples should be presented to help learners understand the rules and strategies.
  c. Instructions should be presented in sequential order.
  d. Sequence needs to be logical and lead systematically to a conclusion.
  e. Rules should provide opportunity for winner(s) to emerge.
  f. Conclusion should be reachable before game becomes boring.
  g. Games should not penalize students who have some kind of handicap.
  h. Accompanying materials should define the game's objective.
  i. Context and format ought to be in good taste.
  j. Objects should not be too complicated (or large) for learners to manipulate.
  k. Context should be well illustrated.
  l. Equipment needs to be strong enough to withstand normal use.
  m. Size and weight should not be cumbersome.
  n. Cost should seem reasonable in terms of educational value.
  o. Learners should be able to transfer learned behavior to a real-life situation.
- Advance preparation.
  a. Pre play with a few students if possible
  b. Check to be sure there are sufficient materials.
  c. Abide by game's recommended number of players whenever possible.
  d. Vary ability levels within each team.
  e. When possible, allow students to choose their own roles and teammates.
  f. Plan time for post game discussion of what has been learned.
- Immediate preparation.
  a. Prepare the room and supplies.
  b. Introduce game briefly, stating purposes.
  c. Review objective if it was introduced earlier.
- Game play
  a. During play, see that things run smoothly.
  b. Do not interrupt, especially to prevent a player(s) from losing.
  c. Be prepared to answer questions about mechanical and structural aspects.
  d. Remain neutral in regard to game strategy.
  e. Encourage participation and question students about decisions and strategies.
  f. Do not be overly concerned with procedural mistakes during play.
  g. Keep the focus on learning, not on winning.
- After the game is over.
  a. Discuss it. As with many other teaching strategies, the largest part of the learning is the discussion that follows.

**Other Related Methodologies:** Simulations, Role Playing, Dramatized Experiences

**References**


Abt, C. C. (1970). Serious games. New York: Viking Compass. (A leading exponent and innovator discusses the use of games.)

Ball, H. (1975). The media specialist looks at instructional games. Audiovisual Journal, 9 (3), 30-31. (Includes some criteria to assist in evaluating and selecting gaming devices.)

Bevis, E. O. (1973). Curriculum building in nursing, a process (pp. 129-136). St. Louis: C. V. Mosby.

Cessario, L. (1987). Utilization of board gaming for conceptual models of nursing. Journal of Nursing Education, 26 (4), 167-169.

Clark, C. C. (1976). Simulation gaming: A new teaching strategy in nursing education, Nurse Educator, 1 (4), 4-9. (An excellent overview of simulation games, their use, and suggestions for the teacher to make. Sources are listed in references on page 9 of the article.)

Cooper, S. (1979). Methods of teaching -- revisited. Games and simulation. Journal of Continuing Education in Nursing, 10 (5), 144.

Courtney, M. E. (1975). Gaming in nursing: A puzzling matter. Journal of Continuing Education in Nursing, 6 (3), 48-50.

Crancer, J., & Maury-Hess, S. (1980). Games: An alternative to pedagogical instruction. Journal of Nursing Education, 19 (3), 45-52.

Davidhizar, R. (1977). Use of simulation games in teaching psychiatric nursing. Journal of Nursing Education, 16 (5), 9-12. (Describes specific games used in teaching psychiatric nursing in a diploma program. Includes role playing as a game.)

Dininny, J. B. (1977). Food rummy, the game of nutrition. Material Child Nursing, 20 (2), 90-91.

Fitzgerald, L., & McCarren, C. (1988). Pursuing accreditation. Nursing and Health Care, 9 (3), 142-145.

Fransecky, R., & Trojanski, J. (1971). A primer on games. AV media and methods, 36-38. (Excellent source on uses and suggestions for uses.)

Kolb, S. (1983). North: A game for teaching concepts of patient care. Nursing Education, 8 (3), 12-15. (Teaches fluid and electrolyte problems of peds patients.)

Morris, L. (1980). Student made, student-played games. American Journal of Nursing, (10), 1816-1818. (Examples of student made games and how they valued and learned from them.)

Rottet, S. M. (1974). Gaming as a learning strategy. Journal of Continuing Education in Nursing, 5 (6), 22-25.

Stanford, G., & Stanford, B. D. (1969). Learning discussion skills through games. New York: Citation Press. (Describes how high school teachers have used games in inner-city and suburban schools.)

Sylvester, M. J. (1974, July/August). Management games: A useful link between theory and practice. Journal of Nursing Administration.

Wolf, M., & Coggins, C. (1987). A workshop for development of simulation games in nursing. Journal of Continuing Education in Nursing 12 (3), 31-34.

# GLOBE

## Definition

*Globe* is an artificial sphere on the surface of which are drawn maps; three-dimensional geographical representation; a model.

## Purposes

- Provides a better representation than a map, because it shows the entire surface.
- Provides a contrived experience.

---

## Advantages

- A globe is three- rather than two-dimensional, a model.
- It can enhance understanding of the flap map.
- It is especially helpful for young learners.

---

## Points to Remember

- Correlate a globe with flap maps.
- Use it with other forms of instruction as a working model.
- Generally, globe should be no smaller than 8 inches in diameter.
- Use globe with bulletin boards, field trips, television, printed matter.
- There are special models of globes -- "write-on," inflatable rubber gloves, plastic, and pulp.
- Students may make their own with chicken wire and paper mache!

## References


Dale, E. (1976). Audiovisual methods in teaching (3rd ed., pp. 223-226, 533-544). New York: Dryden Press, Holt, Rinehart and Winston.

Kinder, J. (1973). Using instructional media (pp. 96-105). New York: D. Van Nostrand.

Harris, R. (1960). The Rand McNally Handbook of Map and Globe Usage. New York: NY: Rand McNally and Company.

Shigematsu, I. & Minowa, M. (1988). Maps that throw light on disease mortality. World Health Forum, 9(3), 444-448.

Viedema, C. (1988). A health and nutrition atlas. World Health, 2-31. NY. (Entire May issue).

## Definition

*Graffiti* is an impromptu writing or drawing on an easily accessible surface that has been prepared. A form of expression.

## Purposes

- Provide an avenue of expression relative to the Affective Domain.
- Provide for communication with peers.
- Provide an opportunity to meet some students' needs for independence and freedom; as well as their desire for prestige, recognition and/or attention.
- Give individuals an escape to the world of fantasy or play.
- Allow for the opportunity to use wit, humor, and creativity.
- Reveal an educational climate -- "where students are at," "what concerns them."
- Allow individuals to express feelings without revealing their identity.

---

## Advantages

- Inexpensive. Simple, easy to use.
- Useful at any age. Promotes unstructured, uncensored, uninhibited communication by individuals (of ideas, fantasies, poems, art, expressions).
- Provides a natural and creative way to relate to one's environment.
- May be especially useful for some groups -- i.e., alienated youth.

## Disadvantages

- Introduces possibility for strong feelings and positions to be taken from highly charged topics and thus may stir up animosity.
- The technique may be extended from the structured educational purpose to defacing of nearby property.
- Anonymity reduces opportunity to work with individuals who may need assistance.

---

## Role of the Teacher

- Prepare area for the graffiti writing or drawing -- wall, poster board, chalkboard, flip chart, or other area.
- Provide tools -- pencils, paints, colored pens, chalk, crayons.
- May provide a stimulus word, phrase, or diagram (may be incomplete).
- Generally, there should be some follow-up with the group (class, course, session)or some way to indicate why the method was used. This may be done by informing the students of the availability of the graffiti board.

**Possible Uses**

- As a stimulus for ideas which have not been assessed earlier and which will then be followed up in some manner appropriate to the level and interest of the learners.
- To encourage discussion.
- In settings where teenagers frequent or where specific groups might benefit (alienated youth, disturbed youth).
- Settings where learners often have much time, such as waiting rooms, or in areas in either in- or out-patient facilities.
- Locations where health care staff (of various levels) are likely to express their concerns that have not been expressed through other and/or previous channels -- i.e., suggestion box.

**References**


Bayer, M. (1980). Saying good bye through graffiti. American Journal of Nursing, 80 (2), 271.

Byre, A., Peven, D., & Schulman, B. (1972). Graffiti therapy. Perspectives in Psychiatric Care, 10 (1), 34-36.

Deiulio, A. M. (1973). Desk top graffiti: Scratching beneath the surface. Journal of Research and Development Education, 7, 100-104. (A study that suggests graffiti as a source of information to be used for evaluating teacher education programs.)

Hitchens, E. (1979). Evaluation: The graffiti technique. Journal of Nursing Education, 18, 46-47.

Kinder, J. S. (1973). Using instructional media (pp. 95-96). New York: Van Nostrand. (A brief section on graffiti as a recognized curriculum activity.)

Robinson, A. (1974). Graffiti: Way-out outlet for patients. RN, 38-39.

## Definition

*Guest Speaker* is an expert who is not a part of the group, who is asked to speak on a specific topic.

## Purposes

- Provide ideas from an expert.
- Introduce new or controversial material (which may not be available in print).
- Add interest and variety.
- Provide a common stimulus for later group discussion or action.
- Provide outside information when a field trip is not possible (or prior to a field trip).

## Selection of a Speaker

- Select carefully based on the objectives of the classes and the qualities of the speaker.
  a. Whenever possible, it is desirable to have someone in the group hear him/her first and report his/her assessment.
  b. Select from those qualified and available on a given subject.
- Sources of speakers
  a. A file of speakers and sources is an invaluable aid to individuals and groups.
  b. <u>You</u> may be the one to initiate this file (from speakers bureaus, professional groups, governmental agencies, community organizations, various councils, etc.).

## Arrange for the Speaker

- Let the speaker know what is expected of him/her.
  a. Provide him/her with the objectives of the group, the exact title (or work it out with him/her), the needs and interests of the members, the program as a whole, and how he/she fits into it, and the expected size of the audience.
  b. Provide the speaker with specifics about:
    1) amount of time he/she will have.
    2) where he/she will appear on the program.
    3) who will do the instruction.
    4) what will follow the presentation-discussion, question period, buzz groups.
  c. Provide him/her with materials:
    1) a copy of the program.
    2) other printed material about the group or which the group will be receiving.
  d. Inquire if he/she has <u>a set fee</u>, or what financial arrangements are expected.
- Confirm all arrangements in writing. Clarify all details necessary. Include arrangements for transportation and housing.
- Obtain information about the speaker:
  a. What he/she wants said about him/her and the subject in the introduction.
  b. If publicity is important, request glossy photograph for advertisement.

   c. Find out what equipment is necessary, or any suggestions for provision of materials (handouts).
- Arrange for someone to meet the speaker upon arrival.
   a. Include all necessary details of transportation, location of buildings and room, names of contact persons, telephone numbers in writing.

**Responsibilities after the Presentation**

- Provide for the necessary transportation remuneration, or detail as previously contracted.
- Include evaluation of the speaker in the file or some other manner which will assist others in future planning or use of this individual.
- A personal letter should be written within a week after the meeting, giving an evaluation of the group's reactions. Press clippings about the speaker may be enclosed.

**Points to Remember**

- Provide suitable physical arrangements: Equipment, seating arrangements.
- Introduce the speaker properly. Introduction should be brief and to the point.
- Provide a question period following the presentation.
   a. The facilitator may conduct the question period, especially if the subject is controversial.
   b. Ask the speaker if he has a preference for who should handle the questions.
- Thank the speaker at the meeting, and later in writing. Provide evaluative comments of both positive and negative nature in the written communiqué.

**References**


Cooper, S. (1982). Our speaker tonight. Journal of Continuing Education in Nursing 13, 40-43.

Knowles, M. S. Informal adult education (pp. 128-130). New York: Association Press. (An older resource which gives briefly the care and treatment of guest speakers.)

Lock, S. (1978). Nice people with no manners. British Medical Journal, 2, 1774-1775.

Markley, K. (1974). Our speaker this evening. Grand Rapids, MI: Zondervan Pub.

# HAIKU

## Definition

*Haiku* is a form of Japanese poetry, borrowed by Western writers, in which a great deal of subtle meaning is expressed in three lines containing five, seven, and five syllables, respectively; used in original writing.

## Purposes

- Provides a creative form of verbal expression.
- Gives the reader a chance to share writer's mood.
- Increases sensitivity to selected topics and issues.

---

**Advantages**

- Haiku is a creative form that is basically simple to use.
- It is versatile -- can be used in a variety of situations.
- It may be used with children and adults.
- It requires no special tools.
- It may be combined with other media.

**Disadvantages**

- Teacher must be knowledgeable to give instructions and assist learners.
- As haiku originated in Japan, the American form is somewhat different in translation, thus making it difficult to locate explicit rules.

---

## Points to Remember

- Allow for co-creation or mood sharing of the reader with the poet.
- Remember that the part "left out" is the most important.
- Haiku should flow smoothly, especially when read aloud.
- A good haiku is capable of being read all in one breath.
- The teacher planning to use haiku would do well to read examples.
- Suggestions to remember:
  a. Haiku have seasonal implications.
  b. Images and phrases should be balanced.
  c. Expression should be natural, not forced.
  d. Haiku depend on emotional effect, not intellectual "point".
- Things to avoid:
  a. Do not put your personal opinion or point of view in the haiku.
  b. Do not humanize nature.
  c. Do not pad with qualifying words, such as adverbs of adjectives, to get the right number of syllables.

**Sample**

Strawberries are ripe
Eat as many as you can
June in a teaspoon.
Lois Leurgans, "Haiku". On the line, June 3, 1973, p. 1.

**References**


Grant, R. E. (1973). Evaluations through haiku. American Journal of Nursing, 73(8), 1339. (Students wrote Haiku in a course in psychiatric nursing.)

Gustafson, M. B. (1979). Methods of teaching-revisited. Try Haiku. Journal of Continuing Education in Nursing, 10(4), 59-60. (Provides suggestions for use in C.E.)

Harr, L. E. (1974). The timbre of Haiku. Instructor, 83(6), 114-115. (The author suggests you know the myths and the facts about haiku before your students begin writing them.)

Los Altos Writers Roundtable. (1966). Borrowed water, A book of American Haiku. Rutland, VT: Charles E. Tuttle Co. (A selection of some 300 poems.)

Taylor, J. A. (1985). Haiku: A form to air feelings about aging. Geriatric Nursing, 6(2), 81-82.

Thomason, N. (1976). Haiku as a media experience. Audiovisual Instruction, 21(3), 62-63. (A report of the combination of haiku with a slide presentation.)

Wyvell, M. L. (1973). American haiku: A classroom experiment. Improving College and University Teaching, 21(2), 135-136. (College students wrote haiku in English classes.)

# HANDOUT

**Definition**

*Handout* is a printed or duplicated material given as "handouts" to learners; such as outlines, job descriptions, bulletins, cartoons, charts, problems, or any number of a variety of materials.

**Purposes**

- Present and organize major points.
- Provide all with the same stimulus or materials.
- Maximize presentation time (minimize need for verbalization and writing).
- Attract, and hold attention.
- Clarify, exemplify, summarize data or concepts.
- Increase individualization (by potential follow-up).
- Create anticipation.

---

**Advantages**

- Allows the learner to have material for review or reference after a presentation.
- All participants have the same information.
- Sustains interest between sessions or to follow-up.
- Provides information that is otherwise difficult to obtain.

**Disadvantages**

- The learning aid is generally a supplement, not a substitute, for oral presentation or demonstration.
- Too many "handouts" tend to distract from the main points of a presentation and/or confuse the learner.
- It is easy to assume that the learners will read and/or reread the materials.
- The presentation may lose its effectiveness if learners are leafing through and reading when they should be listening to the presenter.
- To assist with timing, do not give the learners printed aids at the beginning of the session unless you want to refer to them from the start.
- Caution should be exercised by the presenter that he does not continue talking while materials are circulating.

---

**Responsibilities of Teacher**

- Assess the learner's need for the material, level of content of material, and "fit" with the session objectives.
- Tell the learner why you are giving the material to them.
- Predetermine how to supplement and/or augment the handout -- rather than either reading it verbatim or ignoring it.
- Plan ahead if handouts should be distributed and/or read before, during, or after presentation or discussion.

- Review materials already developed and revise if necessary.
- Preparation of new materials should include consideration of:
  a. Concern for preparing materials which are clear, simple, concise, and complete.
  b. Illustrate as the need requires: itemize, tabulate, outline, use graphs, etc.
  c. Document and obtain permission for use of borrowed materials.
  d. Consider availability of materials to the learner if you do not provide them.
  e. Evaluate cost in terms of time, energy, facilities.
- Creativity is the key to both use of prepared materials and preparation of originals.
- Handouts may be used in a presentation to introduce, outline, organize, review, summarize -- you name it!

**References**


Cooper, S. (1983). Methods of teaching revisited-Handouts and reading lists. Journal of Continuing Education in Nursing, 14, 36-38.

Dale, E. (1969). Audiovisual methods in teaching (3rd ed., pp. 107-135). New York: Dryden Press. (Describe Dale's model or pictorial device in relationship to the process of abstraction.)

McKeachie, W. (1969). Teaching tips (6th ed., pp. 13-14). Lexington, MA: D. C. Health and Co. (A brief section on course outlines.)

Paduano, M. A. (1975). The greening of the classroom. Journal of Nursing Education, 14(2), 20-24. (Describe the creative course introduction used in an A.D. program.)

# HOOK AND LOOP BOARD

## Definition

*Hook and Loop Board* is a substitute for the flannel board that uses a commercial product for the board covering the tape on the objects; a nylon surface containing thousands of tiny nylon loops. "Velcro" is a brand name of hook and loop.

## Purposes

- Attaches objects to a board that would be too heavy for the flannel board.
- Provides quick, easy displays.

---

## Advantages

- The hook and loop board has unusually strong gripping power (5-10 pounds), eliminating slippage of attached objects.
- You can attach three-dimensions, heavy objects such as tools, books, instruments, and parts of machines.
- Three-dimensional display may attract more attention than flat objects.
- The hook and loop board is more useful than flannel board in demonstrating some things.

## Disadvantages

- A hook and loop board is more expensive to make or purchase than a flannel-or felt board.
- Special tape or Velcro has to be placed on the object to be mounted.

---

## How to Make a Hook and Loop Board

- Material may be a substance such as Celotex or other fiberboard that will not warp.
- Purchase hook and loop fabric in desired color at fabric shop.
- Attach fabric to board with wallpaper paste about the consistency of thick gravy.
- Apply fabric to board immediately, with sponge-rubber side down. Be sure fabric is smooth.
- Allow to dry overnight and frame with thick molding for appearance and support.
- Glue 3/8- to 1/2- inch-square pieces of the hook material to backs of objects; allow to dry 10-12 hours.

## Points to Remember

- Do not use too much tape. A 1-inch square of tape, properly applied, will hold 5-10 pounds.
- To keep the surface of the board in good condition, use only Hook 'n Loop tape in displaying objects. Never use pins, staples, or glue directly on the board.

**References**


Dale, E. (1969). Audiovisual methods in teaching (3rd ed., p. 292). New York: Dryden Press, Holt, Rinehart and Winston. (Briefly outlines how to use a hook and loop board.)

Kinder, J. (1973). Using instructional media (p. 157). New York: D. Van Nostrand.

Lange, C. (1976). Developing low-cost teaching materials. Nursing Outlook, 24(10), 614. (Includes the hook and loop board as a low-cost tool a teacher can make.)

Morgan, B., Holmes, G., & Bundy, C. (1976). Methods in adult education (pp. 201-205). Danville, IL: Interstate Printers and Publishers. (Excellent discussion of the advantages and disadvantages of the flannel- or felt board and the hook and loop board. Also tells how to make a hook and loop board.)

# HOUSE OF DELEGATES

## Definition

*House of Delegates Procedure* is a discussion format in which participants follow parliamentary procedure to simulate a House of Delegates session so that current issues come alive.

## Purposes

- Provides an interesting, active format for nurses to address current issues in nursing.
- Requires participants to speak before a group, take a stand on an issue and defend it concisely.
- Increase awareness of both sides of issues to work with peers to plan strategies.

| | |
|---|---|
| **Advantages** | • Creative strategy that adds variety and increases involvement.<br>• Fosters creativity.<br>• Achieves a variety of outcomes. |
| **Disadvantages** | • Requires careful planning and preparation of materials.<br>• May need to review and/or orient learners to parliamentary rules.<br>• Needs a block of time. |

## Points to Remember

- Prepare handouts with information about parliamentary procedure (Robert's or Sturgis). There are a number of excellent books relating to parliamentary procedure and rules of order. Possible areas to be covered are:
  a. a brief summary of general rules for presiding officers,
  b. a classification of various kinds of motions, and
  c. steps in disposing of specific motions.
- Select topics that have a clear pro and con.
- Establish rules for time limits and number of amendments per resolution.
- Determine rules about speaking turns.
- Plan time frames for use within the days of workshop. You may wish to include time for caucus.
- Provide reference lists and materials related to the issue or topic (if necessary).
- Arrange the physical environment -- tables, microphones, etc.
- Determine role of instructors during sessions.

## References


Sullivan, P. and Beelen, J. (1979). Methods of teaching revisited: A format for discussion. Journal of continuing Education in Nursing 10 (5), 15-17.

Morgan, B., Holmes, G., and Brundy, C. (1976). Methods in Adult Education.

# INCIDENT PROCESS

**Definition**

In an *Incident Process* a group is presented with a brief statement of a single event. The group then uses a systematic process to deal with the incident.

**Purposes**

- Develop skill in problem solving.
- Promote inductive thinking.
- Develop generalizations.
- Develop questioning techniques.
- Distinguish fact from inference.

---

**Advantages**

- Specific incident stimulates interest and involvement.
- Allows progression from specific to general, from concrete to abstract.
- Learners are only given the information for which they ask.
- Readily becomes apparent when systematic process is used adequately or inadequately.
- Promotes learning from mistakes or different situations.

**Disadvantages**

- Requires time to develop the incident with all pertinent facts.
- Requires an instructor skilled in use of a systematic process.
- May be confused with a case, which is a compilation of many incidents.
- Requires orientation.
- Students must have adequate background to deal with the incident.

---

**Format**

- Learners are given a brief (three or four sentences) description of an incident.
- Studying the Incident -- each member silently studies the written description of the incident.
- Getting the Facts
  a. leader possesses the facts.
  b. members ask direct questions to bring out facts.
  c. leader gives only facts asked for and avoids answering questions which are judgmental or evaluative.
- Defining the Problem -- may distinguish immediate and long range problem.
- Deciding on Action -- explore possible solutions and select one solution.
- Generalizing -- determine meaning the incident and the process have for subsequent experiences.

**References**

Pigors, P., & Pigors, F. (1955). The incident process. Washington, DC: Bureau of National Affairs.

Pigors, P. (1955). The incident process -- Learning by doing. Adult Education, 3(5), 7.

Pigors, P. (1966). The incident process -- A method of inquiry. Nursing Outlook, 14(10), 48-50.

# INTERVIEW FORUM

## Definition

An *Interview* is a 5-30 minute presentation conducted before an audience in which one or two resource persons respond to systematic questioning by an interviewer about a previously determined topic.

## Purposes

- Present information in a relaxed and informal manner.
- Explore/analyze a problem.
- Clarify issues.
- Introduce/stimulate interest in topic.
- Encourage audience participation following interview.
- Provide, by way of interviewer, a bridge between resource person(s) and audience.
- Obtain knowledge and impressions of an expert or authority.

---

## Advantages

- Brings ideas from expert in organized manner.
- Provides resource person opportunity to avoid delivering a speech.
- Add variety and interest in group discussion.
- Simple technique.

## Disadvantages

- Unable to give a detailed presentation.
- May become series of short speeches if "interviewee" does not give short response.
- Audience needs may be lost.

---

## Responsibilities

Leader

Contact resource person/expert to be interviewed and explain expectations.
Introduce resource person to group members.
Introduce topic.
Interview resource person(s).
Request questions from group.
Summarizes information presented.
Suggests course of action or way to use information.
Evaluate group learning experiences.
May need to plan to physically setup microphones, etc.

Interviewee/Resource Person(s)

Meet with leader prior to class to determine and review expectations.
Prepare relevant material about anticipated questions.
Answer questions from group and leader.
Summarize main issues presented.
Assist in evaluating learning experience.

Group Members

Prepare in advance about topic.
Listen and consider contributions of resource person and leader.
Asks resource person questions related to topic.
Relate meaning to previous learning experiences.
Identify new ideas and determine way to use new information and/or course of action.
Assist in evaluation of the educational activity.

## Suggestions for Selection of Resource Person

- Look for individual who has:
  A. knowledge of the subject.
  B. ability to give brief, direction answers to questions.
  C. ability to respond in an informal manner.

## References


Bergevin, P., Morris, D., & Smith, R. (1963). Adult education procedures (pp. 106-116). New York: Seabury Press.

Canei, R. (no date). Teacher tactics (p. 12). Springfield, OH: Springfield & Clark County J.V.S..

Leypoldt, M. (1967). 40 ways to teach in groups (pp. 77-79). Valley Forge, PA: Judson Press.

# ITERATIVE HYPOTHESIS TESTING

## Definition

*Iterative Hypothesis Testing* is a strategy frequently used in diagnostic reasoning. The person forms diagnostic hypotheses on the basis of minimal clinical data, and these hypotheses create a context for gathering additional relevant data. By an iterative process, hypotheses are either eliminated or confirmed, and those that survive are made progressively more specific.

## Purposes

➢ To teach clinical reasoning.

## Steps in the Strategy

1. Questioning.
2. Justifying.
3. Interpreting and explaining.

## Elaboration of the Steps

- One student has information about a patient and acts as a "data repository."
- This student present a brief description of a patient. (e.g., name, age, reason for seeking nursing and medical care)
- Another student asks a question to produce more data. The student must justify the question before receiving an answer. (e.g., Why asking for the data? What hypothesis is being considered?)
- The group then concurs on the appropriateness of the question.
- The student who is serving as the data repository provides only the information requested.
- The questioner interprets the information elicited by the question and explains how it influences her/his thinking.
- This serial questioning, justifying, and interpreting process continues until all relevant data has been extracted, all issues discussed, a diagnosis is achieved, or time runs out.

## References

Kassirer, J. (1983). Teaching clinical medicine by iterative hypothesis testing: Let's preach what we practice. New England Journal of Medicine, 309 (15), 921-923.

Elstein, A., Shulman, L., & Sprafka, S. (1978). Medical problem solving. Cambridge, MA: Harvard University Press.

## Definition

*Jeopardy* is a television game whose format can be used for teaching.

## Purposes

- Use a creative teaching strategy to motivate students and add interest and variety for the teacher.
- Learn new knowledge, apply concepts, and review information.

---

**Advantages**

- Adds interest.
- Especially useful if material seems dry, boring, or repetitious.
- Can be used for any number of learners (2-30+).
- Once developed, can be used repeatedly.
- Many areas are content appropriate, but not all are (i.e., grief).

**Disadvantages**

- Both teacher and students need to be familiar with the format.
- Developing the initial game can be time consuming.
- Some may see it as less that a serious educational endeavor.

---

## Points to Remember

- Determine goal for the game (pretest, posttest, tension-reliever, exam review).
- Determine how much time you need to play (verses the actual time you have).
- Develop objectives to cover the content you wish to test or review.
- Select content, being sure it is appropriate to the format.
- Develop questions for the teams to answer, list them according to categories and $ value. You may wish to have all the ones in Category A on one sheet, etc.
- Rehearse with colleagues to check out your categories and become comfortable with the game, and determine the appropriate time frame.
- Evaluate and revise prior to use with the students.

## Implementation

- Prior to use of the game, you need to draw the game on flip chart -- unless you have prepared a more permanent game board. List categories on the horizontal axis and values vertically.
- Determine the two teams.
- Arrange for time-keeping, either with opposing team or other designate.

- According to the TV format, the question is in the form of an answer (or statement), and the answer is given in a form of a question. Responses are made by "What is...."
- It is nice to have prizes -- candy, stickers, or other items.
- You may wish to tape and use some of the actual TV music* from the program.

**References**


Cooper, S. (1989). Creative teaching strategies. Journal of Continuing Education in Nursing, 20, 95-96.

Patten, B. (1989). Brief: When to place your staff in "Jeopardy" -- A CPR teaching strategy. Journal of Continuing Education in Nursing 20, 136-137.

*Trebek, A., & Barsochini. (1994). The Jeopardy book. (Harper Perennial, pb $12.95).
(The history of the show, rules of play, backstage anecdotes by host Trebek, and a copy of the theme music. Plus 100 pages of answers and questions, laid out in "Jeopardy" board form.)

# KAMISHIBAI

**Definition**

*Kamishibai* is a box theater used to show a series of flat pictures; (Kami = paper, shibai = drama)

**Purposes**

- ➢ Accompany a narrative with pictures that move.

---

**Advantages**

- Inexpensive, since locally available materials may be used.
- Familiar form for many (old method, originated in Japan)
- Simple to make and operate.
- Portable, easy to transport.
- Adaptable, may be ethnic/culture specific, and adapted to local situations.
- Students (individuals or groups) may prepare (and use) the box theater and drawings.

**Disadvantages**

- May be difficult to see if group is small.
- Requires some equipment and some basic drawing ability.
- May be most appreciated by elementary age learners.
- May not be viewed as educational; since has been used to entertain and sell merchandise.

---

**Points to Remember**

- Equipment consists of box with front stage opening and side opening for pictures. Pictures are on cards or rolls of paper. Stand is optional.
- Carton or box may be used for the theater.
- Discarded materials may be used. (i.e., old curtain rods, bamboo poles, rollers)
- Newsprint may be used for pictures.
- Narrative which correlates may be placed on back of preceding picture.
- Use of story board may help in planning. (See Kemp below or Story board guidelines)

**References**

Kemp, J. (1963). Planning and producing audio visual materials(3rd ed., pp. 52-54). New York: Thomas Y. Crowell.

Pampiglione, S. (1980). Kamishibai. WHO Chronicle, 34(10), 386-387. (Contains model and suggestions for making one).

# LAMINATION

## Definition

*Lamination* is the process of coating visual media with thin layers of tough, mylar film to make them airtight.

## Purposes

- Provide permanent protective covering bond of dry surfaces.
- Protect, preserve, and add usefulness to charts, maps, drawings, pictures, clippings, documents, etc.
- Render visuals airtight, waterproof, and smear proof.

---

**Advantages**

- Protect materials from dirt and moisture.
- Not complicated, messy or difficult.
- Useful on a variety of materials, surfaces, and objects.
- Less expensive than replacing visuals.
- Increases types of uses for a visual.
- Makes them more durable for repeated use.

**Disadvantages**

- Some items, such as a color photograph, can be damaged by high temperatures required.
- Cost of commercial laminating may be expensive, but worth it.

---

## Types of Laminating

Cold Laminating: Hand, clipboard, machine (cold acetate laminator).
Heat Laminating: Four different types of machines. (Heat acetate, acetate pouch, dry mounting press, and thermocopy machine laminator).

## Points to Remember

- Surfaces need to be dry and clean.
- When machines are used, follow directions closely.
- Body oils from handling materials (or moisture) can cause non/partial adhesion.
- When in doubt as to use of cold or hot lamination, read directions or inquire before proceeding.
- Problems with bubbles, wrinkles, and stress lines are due to non or partial adhesion.
- Some matte acetate will accept pencil, ball-point pen , and typewriter notations.
- Follow instructions for laminating kits you purchase.

## Definition

*Learning Fair* is an educational experience where a variety of ideas, demonstrations, and games available to learners. Also known as "skills fairs."

## Purposes

- Provide a different approach to sharing and learning.
- "Loosen" people up so they recognize all conceivable learning -- emotional, physical, intellectual, mystical.
- Provide opportunity for learners of a variety of ages and interests to come together as participants/innovators.
- Individualize instruction.
- Provide learning experiences that are fun, open-ended, and exploratory.
- Provide maximum direct action involvement.
- Provide for learners to teach peers.
- Stimulate curiosity about group members' ideas/products.
- Vicarious learning.
- Provides for self-paced learning.

---

**Advantages**

- Provides for involvement of students and teachers.
- Gives opportunity for demonstration of creativity (process and products).
- Especially useful in teaching the affective and psychomotor domains.
- Can provide support to adults and older children when they "open up."
- Gives opportunity to identify resources within a group.
- If time limits are a part of the activity an additional outcome may be learning to be concise.
- Can offer a variety of learning experiences in one learning activity.

**Disadvantages**

- Requires planning, organizing and adequate space.
- May require additional equipment, materials, and faculty time to prepare learners and the facility/setting.
- May be perceived as "only for small children."

---

**Responsibilities**

Teacher:

a. Provide learners with clear objectives and responsibilities for the experience.
b. Provide clear instructions to time, place, course of action.
c. Make necessary arrangements for materials, equipment, and procedures.
d. May be offered as an optional activity or approach.

Learner:

a. Use objectives provided.
b. Bring a specific "something" to share in the time provided.

**Other Related Methodologies:** Learn-o-Rama, Skills Fair.

**Procedural Sample:**

Title: Learning Fair

Objectives:

To select an aspect of one teaching experience to share with classmates.
To identify resources within peer group.
To identify a wide variety of approaches for each component of the teaching-learning process.
To experience the learning fair approach.

| Groups: | I -- Room 34 | II -- Room 35 | II -- Room 36 |
|---|---|---|---|
| | 1. Mark | 1. Chrissy | 1. Susan |
| | 2. Jeanne | 2. Judy | 2. Marie |
| | 3. Brano | 3. Donna | 3. Christopher |
| | 4. Tracey | 4. Colleen | 4. Diane |

Schedule:

11:15-11:25

a.) Announcements and Orientation to Procedure.

11:25-11:40

a.) Each group meet in room identified.
b.) First person on list present for four minutes.
c.) At sound of bell, all but first person on each list move to next room.
d.) First person on list will present four times until all groups have participated.

11:40-11:55

a.) Everyone return to original identified room.
b.) Second person on list present for four minutes.
c.) Proceed in same fashion.

11:55-12:10
  a.) Everyone return to original assigned room.
  b.) Third person on list present for four minutes.
  c.) Proceed in same fashion.
12:15-12:30
  a.) All return to Room 33 to summarize.

**References**

Brady, L. (1985). Faculty continuing education: Teaching methods. Journal of Continuing Education in Nursing, 16, 26-28.

Sands, S. (1972, Dec.). Learning fair. Saturday Review, 38-41.

# LECTURE

**Definition**

*Lecture* is a method of teaching by which the instructor gives an oral presentation of facts or principles, the class usually being responsible for note taking; usually implies little or no class participation by such means as questioning or discussion during the class period.

**When it is Appropriate to Use**

- Large classes.
- Direct learners to large quantity of material in a limited time.
- Interpretation of facts and ideas, especially when complicated or difficult to comprehend.
- Subject is not adequately covered by easily accessible materials.
- To inspire and stimulate.

---

**Advantages**

- Large numbers may be accommodated, therefore, economical.
- Usually the simplest way of presenting unfamiliar material.
- Able to convey what isn't available readily.
- Able to present latest information that may not be published yet.
- Requires a minimum of equipment and/or facilities.
- Efficient use of time (and faculty).
- Less time is needed than to discover a principle.
- Teacher maintains primary control.

**Disadvantages**

- Over stress on acquisition of information and lower levels of learning.
- Lack of learner participation, learner is able to be more passive.
- Difficult to adjust for individual differences.
- Appeals to one sense only -- hearing.
- May give limited viewpoint on controversial material.
- May require concentration for too long a period of time.
- Difficult to check for comprehension, limited feedback.

---

**Variations or Combinations**

- Lecture supplemented with films, slides, videos, overheads, or other audiovisual materials.
- Lecture-discussion, e.g., lecture more informal, part of time is planned for clarification and questions.
- Lecture-demonstration, e.g. include "how to" demonstration in presentation.
- Lecture-recitation, e.g., following the lecture, students answer and/or ask questions to clarify their understandings.

## Points to Remember

- Prepare thoroughly.
- Caution with the number of facts and ideas included -- and total amount of content.
- Organization must be systematic.
- Supplement with illustrations, stories, objects, drawing pictures.
- Use clear, forceful language.
- Individualize content to the teacher -- put self into it!
- Use humor and wit.
- In delivery be concerned for pacing, speed, time for notes, voice quality.
- Note taking -- plan for it by including outlines, handouts, use of blackboard.
- Plan for reaction from students.

## References


Blauch, L. E. (1945). Teaching in colleges and universities (pp. 129-146). Indianapolis, IN: American Association of Dental Schools. (An old, but complete discussion of the lecture method.)

Borden, R. C. (1935). How to communicate ideas. (From the book by Borden, Public Speaking As Listeners Like It. Harper & Row). (Booklet on speechmaking.)

Gagne, R. (1965). The conditions of learning (pp. 288-289). New York: Holt, Rinehart & Winston. (Brief discussion of recitation class.)

Gaut, D., & Blainey, C. (1982). The lecture approach to teaching nursing-method or habit? Nursing & Health Care, 3, 73-77.

Gustafson, M. (1987). Get going! Get done! Instructions and conclusions for your class. Journal of Continuing Nursing Education, 18(3), 103-104.

McKeachie, W. J. (1969). Teaching tips: A guide book for the beginning college teacher (6th ed.). Lexington, Mass: D.C. Health & Company. (Gives a sketchy outline of what is important in considering use of the lecture, but gives findings from several research studies on the values of the method.)

Puleo, Sister M. P. (1968). Comparison of on-the-job and at-home use of programmed instruction and the lecture method in an in-service education program. Nursing Research, 17(4), 356-360.

Van Hoozer, H., Brink, P., & Oppligen, R. (1989). The effects of overhead transparency design on retention, recall, and application of data analysis content. Journal of Nursing Education, 28(4), 181-187.

Bloom, B. S., et al. (1956). Taxonomy of educational objectives, handbook I: Cognitive domain. New York: David McKay Company, Inc.

Budd, R. (1969). A picture is still worth more than a thousand words. Nursing Outlook, 17(15), 48-49.

Ruhland, F. R. (1973). Telelecture? Try it, you'll like it. Journal of Continuing Education in Nursing, 4(2), 14-18. (The author explains very clearly her experiences and value of this form of lecture.)

Weaver, R.II. (1986). Using interactive images in the lecture hall. Education Horizons, 64(4), 180-185.

## LESSON PLAN

**Definition**

*Lesson Plan* is a teaching outline of the important points of a lesson arranged in the order in which they are to be presented; may include objectives, points to be made, questions to ask, references to materials, assignments, etc.

**Purposes**

- Gives direction for instruction.
- Stimulates creative teaching.
- Gives a student who is learning to teach, the opportunity to see progress over time.
- Assures consistency and thoroughness in both lesson and course.

---

**Advantages**

- A lesson plan ensures completeness and thoroughness.
- It increases teacher's self-confidence.
- It allows critique of plan by peers and/or instructors prior to teaching.
- It allows the mentor to assess how individual class fits into course and overall curriculum.
- Plans are available for a substitute teacher or for future use.

**Disadvantages**

- Plan is time-consuming and a lot of work.
- It may inhibit a of spontaneity.
- Teaching from a lesson plan may become repetitive, "rote," and uncreative.

---

**Essential Parts of any Plan**

- Assessment
  a. "Fit" of class into course, unit, and program.
  b. Learners' level, readiness, motivation, learning needs, learning style.
  c. Facilities.
  d. Time available.
- Planning
  a. Learner objectives (may be stated behaviorally, may reflect domains and levels)
  b. Personal objectives (may be stated similarly to learner objectives)
  c. Approach determined from alternatives of teaching methods and learner experiences; chosen because of rationale based on learning theory and principles of learning.
  d. Content planned and differentiated as to essential content; rationale based on learning theory.
  e. Evaluation included in plans, may utilize pre- and post-testing.

- Development
  a. Introduction.
  b. Sequence of content -- may include activities, strategies, marginal notes to remind teacher of points or questions, time schedule, or other reminders as to the general progression of the allotted time.
  c. Summary.
- Evaluation
  a. Specific to evaluation of learning, teaching, or teacher, or a combination of the three.
  b. Criteria and means for evaluation -- tool(s) may be original or borrowed.
  c. Self-evaluation.
- Bibliography
  a. Content or topic related.
  b. Methodology or teaching strategies.

**Points to Remember**

- Teacher may wish to follow predetermined format provided, or create their own lesson plan.
- Other sources of lesson plans may be plans written by other teachers.
- After determining the basic aspects and a plan that is inclusive and convenient, experiment.
- You may wish to keep a file, being sure to date the plan and the update or revisions.

**References**

Conklin, K. (1975). Why are lesson plans always incomplete? Educational Forum, 40(1), 67-72. (Describes the dynamic, individual, changing nature of the lesson plan, not the lack of need for plans.)

Emo, D. (1977). Preparing a lesson plan. Imprint, 24(3), 53. (While a nursing student, the author suggested some ideas for lesson plan writing.)

Jeffries, D. (1966). Lesson planning and lesson teaching. Titusville, NJ: Home and School Press. (This 581 -- page book contains an exhaustive discussion of lesson plans.)

## LIMERICK

### Definition

*Limerick* is a humorous, nonsense poem of five anapestic lines; where lines, 1, 2 and 5 are three feet and rhyme and lines 3 and 4 are two feet and rhyme. Light verse form appeals through ridiculous humor, wordplay, and bouncing anapestic rhythm.

### Purpose

- Humorous, amusing form.
- Powerful way to express oneself.

### Construction Pattern

- 2 amphibrachic trimeters.
- 2 anapestic dimeters.
- First line repeated in last with only minor variations of syntax or vocabulary.

### Points to Remember

- Any verse that does not follow that pattern, however clever it may be, is simply not a limerick, it is a verse.

### References


Gustafson, M. (1993). Lessons from Dr. Seuss? Health World, 5 (3), 14-15.

Lear, N. (1980). A book of nonsense. New York: Metropolitan Museum of Art & Viking Press.

Livingston, M. (1991). Lots of limericks. New York: McElderry Books.

Parrott, E. (1990). The Penquin book of limericks. New York: Viking Press.

Seuss, Dr. (1996) You're only old once! A book for obsolete children. New York: Random House (or any other of his books).

## Definition

*Magic* is having unusually distinctive qualities resembling the supernatural; producing startling and amazing effects-tricks, illusions, and sleight of hand.

## Purposes

- Educational use is to teach or change behavior.
- Adds interest to verbal presentations.
- Attract attention.
- Motivate learners and direct learning tasks.

---

## Advantages

- Universal appeal.
- Intrigues all ages.
- Evokes surprise, delight, or astonishment.
- May be made culture specific.
- Is largely an unused method.
- May elicit audience participation.

## Disadvantages

- The magic or magician may overshadow the lesson.
- Some skill is required in performing.
- The use of magic or tricks may have a negative connotation in some areas/cultures.

---

## Points to Remember

- Relationship of magic to learning objective needs careful planning.
- Message should be clear and simple.
- "Magician" needs to practice.
- Enhancement is likely if locally available materials and known circumstances are used.
- Discussion and audience participation should be a planned part.
- Magicians' Code:
  a. Don't reveal the secret of a trick, even to your best friend.
  b. Don't perform the same trick twice before the same audience.
  c. Don't do any trick for friends until you have practiced it.
  d. Don't interfere with others when they do magic.

**References**

Becker, G. (1978). It's magic. Teacher, 95(7), 53.

Becker, G. (1979, April). The magician of health. Salubritas, 3(2), 1.

Van Dokkum, W. (1978). The application of magic as an audio-visual in nutrition education. Cajanus, 11(4), 235-241.

Windley, C. (1976). Put a little magic in your room! Instructor, 86(4), 70-72.

Windley, C. (1976). Teaching and learning with magic (p. 13). Washington, DC: Acropolis Books.

# MANUAL

**Definition**

*Manual* is a book, booklet, or leaflet indicating the use of materials or describing operation or indication for equipment and/or concepts.

**Purposes**

- Instruct in matters of procedure or policy.
- Assist teacher in planning, through manual that accompanies a textbook.
- Assist learner in orientation.
- Prepare individuals for group discussion.

---

**Advantages**

- Provide the most current information available on policy and procedure.
- Provide all individuals with the same information about requirements for a procedure or psychomotor skill.
- Saves instructors time when learners study prior to class session.
- Provides learners with opportunity to prepare at their own time and pace.
- Supplements verbal instruction given in class.

**Disadvantages**

- Lengthy reading assignments not suitable due to technical language.
- Due to psychomotor skill requirements, it may be necessary to supplement reading of the manual with discussion.

---

**Suggestions for Preparation of Manual**

- You may wish to review other manuals for examples.
- Strive for conciseness and clarity in instructions.
- Use technical language cautiously.
- Using and stating the principles that guide the use of the instruction is both appropriate and meaningful in some manuals.
- Seek help of script writers and visual graphic experts.
- May wish to include complete addresses of manufacturers of some products or equipment.
- Pretest manual with both novice and expert before final publication.
- Be sure the date of development is clearly indicated.
- Plan periodic revision to maintain information that is up-to-date.

**Points to Remember**

- Select portions of the manual pertinent to your topic, if the entire manual is not appropriate.
- Explain to learners the purpose of the manual and how to use it.
- Supply reasons and rationale for stated policies and procedures.
- Encourage clarification of any aspects considered confusing or difficult.
- Apply manual information to specific situations and encourage immediate application in this work setting.
- Plan for evaluation feedback.
- When appropriate, plan for observation of psychomotor skill that was taught in the manual.

**Other Related Methodologies:** Pamphlet, Handbook.

**References**


Brown, J. W., Lewis, R. B., & Harcleroad, F. L. (1964). AV instruction, materials and methods (2nd ed.). New York: McGraw-Hill.

California State Department of Employment. More learning in less time -- Manuals. Sacramento, CA. n.d.

Fleishman, E. A. (1964). Examiner's manual for the basic fitness tests. Englewood Cliffs, NJ: Prentice-Hall. (Example of manual).

King, E. M., Wieck, L., & Dyer, M. (1981). Illustrated manual of nursing techniques (2nd ed.). Philadelphia: Lippincott. (Example of Nursing manual).

Steel, J. L. (1982). What manual? Getting policies and procedures on the line. Nursing Management, 13(3), 43-46.

Dowling, M. (1988). How to make manuals for health workers. World Health, 9(3), 414-419.

Rubenson, B. (1988). Health teaching made easier: How to create a manual. Contact, 105, 1-6.

# MAPS

## Definition

*Map* is a representation of a surface or some part of it, showing the relative size and position according to some given scale. Any two-dimensional depiction. Also called "flat map." A concept may also be represented in a map. Maybe called "conceptual map" or mind map.

## Purposes

- Provides students with knowledge of both relative and exact positions of political units, land masses, and water areas.
- Furnishes information about areas, distances, directions, shapes, sizes, and relationships.
- Adds meaning to straight descriptive material.
- Stimulates inquisitiveness about people, places, and geography.

---

**Advantages**

- A map shows geographical or conceptual relationship in two dimensions.
- It explains facts that might otherwise be complex, dry, or meaningless.
- It makes abstract names concrete.
- It delineates geographical locations in symbols, words, and drawings.
- It can be a source of enlightenment and enrichment.
- Inexpensive maps may be prepared by teachers and students.

**Disadvantages**

- Every flat map contains distortions because it presents our spherical earth on a flat surface.
- A map may omit details and condense information.
- It requires some basic reading skills and understanding of symbols.

---

## Types of Maps

Physical-political. The most common one shows political boundaries, mountains, cities, rivers.
Pictorial-statistical. Uses pictures or dots to show location of important data for relationships.
Relief. Generally three-dimensional representations, showing earth's surface, features, elevations, irregularities, and topography.
Outline. A skeleton with little more than boundary markings. Students place information on it.
Mind map. Shows an outline of concepts and ideas.
Atlas. A collection of maps bound together.

**Other Related Methodologies**: Globe.

## Points to Remember

- You need to teach stages of map reading and meaning of symbols.
- It may be helpful to point out important features.
- Check for lighting and height of mounted wall maps.
- Uses are many, ranging from orientation to a facility to demographic studies and international aspects of health care.
- Sources of maps might be commercial, government agencies, nonprofit agencies, and societies.
- Maps should be stored carefully -- small ones files and large ones rolled or folded.

## Standards for Judging Maps

- Visibility
- Detail
- Scale
- Symbols
- Color
- Accuracy
- Appropriateness to level of learner
- Point of view
- Durability
- Accessibility

## References


Dale, E. (1976). Audiovisual methods in teaching (3rd ed., pp. 223-226, 533-544). New York: Dryden Press, Holt, Rinehart and Winston.

Kinder, J. (1973). Using instructional media (pp. 96-105). New York: D. Van Nostrand.

Harris, R. (1960). The Rand McNally Handbook of Map and Globe Usage. New York: NY: Rand McNally and Company.

Shigematsu, I. & Minowa, M. (1988). Maps that throw light on disease mortality. World Health Forum, 9(3), 444-448.

Viedema, C. (1988). A health and nutrition atlas. World Health, 2-31. NY. (Entire May issue).

# MNEMONICS

## Definition

*Mnemonics* are short verbal devices that encode long series of facts in formulas or ways that make them easy to recall.

## Purposes

- Assist memory and recall.
- Add interest.
- Enable information to be connected.

---

**Advantages**

- Anyone of any age can compose them.
- Teachers may devise specific ones for their own use.
- Useful in any discipline.
- There are several collections available.

**Disadvantages**

- There are folklore variations.
- They may be viewed as nonsense and therefore deemed to be less valuable.

---

## Forms

- Acrostic like sentence.
- Jingle mnemonics (rhythm and rhyme).
- Acronym -- each letter of a word stands for name or a piece of information.

## References


A Dictionary of Mnemonics. (1972). London: eye Methuen Ltd.

Atkinson, R. (1975). Mnemotechnics in second language learning. American Psychologist, 30, 821-828.

Belleza, F. (1981). Mnemonic devices: Classification, characteristics, and criteria. Review of Educational Research, 51, 247-275.

Biggers, V. (1992). Codes for a code: Easy ACLS memory aids. American Journal of Nursing, 92, 56-61.

Brett, Sunib. (Ed) (1981). The Faber Book of useful verse. London: Faber & Faber Ltd.

Hall, J., & Fuson, K. (1986). Presentation rates in experiments on mnemonics: A methodological note. Journal of Educational Psychology, 78, 233-234.

Jamieson, D., & Schimpf, M. (1980). Self-generated images are more effective mnemonics. Journal of Mental Imagery, 6, 25-30.

Pressley, M., Levin, J. & Delaney, H. (1982). The mnemonic keyboard method. Review of Educational Research, 52, 61-91.

Suid, M. (1981). Demonic mnemonics. Belmont, CA: David S. Lake.

# MODELS

**Definition**

*Model* is a scaled representation, which may be equal in size, smaller, or larger than original.

**Purposes**

- Presents a visual representation of an object.
- Adds interest and meaning to displays and exhibits.
- In demonstrations, generates interest and stimulates thought.
- Clarifies parts and actions of objects that move.
- Demonstrates relationships of parts to the whole.

---

**Advantages**

- A model shows clearly and quickly "how" and "why" something works.
- It permits close-up observation, investigation, and analysis.
- It provides direct contact with actual objects.
- It is useful for all age groups.
- It is easy to use in explanation.
- It may be used repeatedly.
- Teacher and students may make inexpensive models from a variety of materials.
- Large simulation devices have proven effective in teaching skills (airline pilots, driver education).
- Some models may be purchased ready-made or ready-cut.

**Disadvantages**

- Oversimplification is sometimes a danger.
- Students may get erroneous concepts of size and complexity.
- Commercial models are often costly to purchase.
- Models may require large storage space, special atmospheric conditions, or extreme care of handling.

---

**Types of Models**

Solid. Used for recognition of external features (puppets, engines, cars).
Cross section or cutaway. Shows internal structure (anatomical models, machines).
Construction models. Put together part by part (human torso, human skeleton).
Working models. Show how machines work.

**Points to Remember**

- Select or construct model based on true impression. Use accurate, most recent revision of a form, and supply sensory experiences as fully as possible (proper sound, for example).
- Show at appropriate time.
- Relate model's operation to settings and situations in real life.
- Point out what to observe, and why. Show motion when it is involved.
- Use model interestingly; add anecdotes and historical data.
- Place model in convenient location for all to see.
- Allow students to handle and manipulate model.
- Encourage examination, question asking, and generalization.
- Put unrelated models out of sight so they don't confuse students.
- Clarify purpose of model.
- Provide practice session if appropriate. Include instructor, if necessary, to explain and clarify.
- Encourage student production of models.

**Other Related Methodologies:** Mockups, Moulage, Cutaways, Specimens, Equipment, Mannequin.

**References**

Kinder, J. S. (1973). Using instruction media (pp. 159-161). New York: D. Van Nostrand.

Schweer, J. E. (1972). Creative teaching in clinical nursing (pp. 186-187). St. Louis: C.V. Mosby.

deTornyay, R. (1971). Strategies for teaching nursing (pp. 26-28). New York: John Wiley & Sons.

# MOULAGE

**Definition**

*Moulage* is to reconstruct a model or cast made directly from any portion of the body, application of make-up to simulate injuries.

**Purposes**

- Provide realism for clinical simulation scenarios (various injuries may be simulated: lacerations, abrasions, bruises, fractures, burns, sucking chest wounds, etc.)

---

**Advantages**

- Experiences are more realistic
- There are inexpensive substitutes available which can be prepared and used.

**Disadvantages**

- Time is required to gather, clean up and store materials
- It may be difficult to determine or prepare some substitutes
- Some products (both commercial or "homemade" may be harmful to individual's skin, clothing, and furnishings).

---

**Points to Remember**

- Apply moulage in air-conditioned and very cool environment.
- Allow sufficient time to prepare each "victim".
- Prepare well in advance of class or drill.
- Essential supplies and specifically how to prepare appear in the Hindman articles below.

**Other Related Methodologies:** Simulation

**References**


Hindman, D. (1988). Moulage: Setting up a basic kit. Journal of Emergency Nursing 14, 316-317.

Hindman, D. (1988). The application of moulage. Journal of Emergency Nursing 14, 379-382.

Naeve, R. (1989). Pictures in the round: Moulage and modes in medicine. Journal of Audiovisual Media in Medicine, 12, 80-84.

Stenberg, J. (1987). Teaching IV therapy: Getting closer to reality. Nurse Educator, 12, 33-35.

# MULTIPLE STUDENT ASSIGNMENT

## Definition

*Multiple Student Assignment* is a "Team Learning" instructional method in which a group of 2-4 students learn together by being assigned to one patient or project. Each student has specialized role and a specialized set of objectives for the experience. The roles are alternated periodically so that each student has an opportunity to experience different aspects of the total patient care or project. (deLorey).

## Roles

The Doer -- applies theoretical knowledge to the situation and carries out the plan of action developed by the group.
Information Gatherer -- collects pertinent information from all possible sources.
Observer -- observes interactions among patient, student, and team. Provides support and constructive criticism for the doer. (Generally considered the most difficult role).

---

**Advantages**

- Students learn to look at intellectual aspects as well as psychomotor aspects of an assignment or project.
- Each student is able to focus on one circumscribed aspect while still contributing to overall plan of action.
- Provides for both direct and vicarious learning.
- May provide for more realistic self evaluation as students are able to observe and share with a peer.
- Problem-solving can be utilized more frequently at greater depth.
- Experiences in group process and collaboration are provided; students learn together as well as learn to work together.
- Decreases number of patients necessary for meaningful clinical experience.
- Provides immediate peer feedback based on current observations resulting in early identification of appropriate behaviors and errors in performance.

**Disadvantages**

- Inadequate guidance from the instructor may result in confusion and/or fragmented learning and patient care.
- Often there is initial reluctance or suspicion about this method on the part of both students and staff. Conversely, patients tend to accept the method willingly. (deLorey).

---

## Teacher's Role

- Provide orientation and explanation to students and staff.
- Carefully select patients. Determine how patient situation will provide opportunities for each student in group to meet objectives.
- Provide adequate guidance to maximize benefits of this approach.
- Be available as a resource person.
- Prevent a student from submerging him/herself in activities alone.
- Provide frequent opportunity for all involved to express their feelings about this method.
- Help the team reflect on their experience.
- Provide sufficient number of experiences with the same team members so that both students and teacher become aware of growth within the team.

## References


deLorey, P. (1972). Multiple assignment: Rehearsal for practice. American Journal of Nursing, 72(2), 292-295. (An excellent description of the strategy as well as the responsibilities and difficulties of all participants in the multiple assignment method.)

Fugate, T., & Rebeschi, L. (1992). Dual assignment: An alternative clinical teaching strategy. Nurse Educator, 17, 14-16.

Galeener, J. (1966). Providing more meaningful clinical experience through groups or multiple student assignments. Journal of Nursing Education, 5(2), 29. (A brief, general description of the multiple assignment method as used in a junior college setting.)

Glanville, C. (1971). Multiple assignment as an approach to clinical teaching in pediatric nursing. Nursing Research, 20(3), 237-244. (This study was designed to investigate the effectiveness of multiple student assignments in pediatric nursing in a baccalaureate program. Eleven 3rd year students participated, 6 in the experimental group and 5 in the control group. The analysis of data indicated no significant differences in the outcome of student learning between the students taught by multiple assignments and those taught by the traditional method.)

Hatroch, B. (1969). Multiple student assignments. Nursing Outlook, 17(11), 40-42. (A good overview of the purpose, the roles involved and the difficulties of multiple assignments as used in an associate degree program.)

VanDenBerg, E. L. (1976). The multiple assignment: An effective alternative for laboratory experiences. Journal of Nursing Education, 15(3), 3-12. (A study of 22 students in an A.D. program, testing the efficacy of both the traditional and multiple assignment approaches.)

# MUSIC

## Definition

*Music* is the art and science of the creation and production of aesthetically appealing tonal sequences and combinations.

## Purposes

- Utilize an art form for educational purposes.
- Connect known themes in a non-educational setting with a specific educational objective.
- Provides interest and flexibility in approaching concepts and issues.

---

## Advantages

- Well known lyrics are often familiar (popular songs, classical music).
- Readily available and inexpensive -- may be borrowed or purchased locally.
- Adds variety when another vehicle is combined with teaching method.
- Versatile. Can approach a topic from a variety of perspectives.
- May introduce controversial or contradictory issues and opinions (i.e., ethical, social, or political concerns).
- Flexible in amount of time required (i.e., from brief segment used to introduce and/or set tone to a detailed discussion of meanings and implications.)
- Music can promote retention of information and ideas.

## Disadvantages

- May be difficult to obtain music and lyrics specifically related to a topic or issue.
- Students may wish to discuss the effect of the music which is different from the teacher's objectives.
- If recording quality is poor, it may detract rather than add.

---

## Points to Remember

- Teacher needs to be clear and share objective(s) for using the music.
- Need to remember that music tends to evoke feeling. Music may be associated with a previous experience of the learner.
- Teacher needs to listen to entire piece before using all or part.
- If listeners are unfamiliar with lyrics or point being made -- may need time to hear more than once.

- ➢ Sometimes it may be helpful to have accompanying words.
- ➢ Study questions and written instructions on what to listen for or what to consider may be helpful.
- ➢ Teacher should be sure of playback quality and how to work equipment (cassette, phonograph, CD).

**References**


Cooper, B. (1979). Popular music: A creative teaching resource. Audiovisual Instruction, 24(3), 37-43. (Defines popular music and discusses how it might be used as a teaching resource. Lists teaching approaches using popular music and some concepts and issues to be investigated.)

Herth, K. (1978). The therapeutic use of music. Supervisor Nurse, 9(9), 22-23. (A nursing coordinator on a 40 bed medical/surgical unit of a general hospital suggests uses in clinical practice.)

Meeks, L. (1977). The role of spiritual health in achieving high level wellness. Health Values: Achieving High-Level Wellness, 1(5), 222-224. (Suggests use of poems and music to share one's belief system.)

Werner, D., & Bower, B. (1982). Helping health workers learn. Palo Alto, CA: Hesperian Foundation.

# MYTH

## Definition

*Myth* is an imaginative explanation or interpretation by man of himself or of objects and events in nature. (Chief characters were deities, with heroes, common mortals, and animals in subordinate roles).

## Characteristics

- Based on primitive belief in animated world and animism; animated nature taken for granted.
- Have become sacred literature when written.
- Culture hero is presented to listener as a figure he ought to emulate.
- Pessimistic, ending nearly always tragic.
- May express inner conflict in symbolic form.
- There are various classifications.

## Purposes

- Ancient:
  a) explain scientific symbols
  b) explain religious nature and philosophy of life. Truth.

{ Modern:
  a) orient and give perspective
  b) key to literary allusion.

---

**Advantages**

- Universal
- Similar to animal fables, hero tales, folk tales and fairy tales.
- Assist in understanding beliefs.

**Disadvantages**

Requires wide knowledge of source material.
Need thorough understanding of the hero and his/her times if going to adopted.

---

## Components of A Typical Myth

- preliminary situation
- initial incident
- rising action (via steps)
- climax
- falling action
- conclusion

**<u>Other Related Methodologies</u>:** Fable, Fairy Tale, Folk Tale, Legend.

## References


Bettelheim, B. (1977). The uses of enchantment, the meaning and importance of fairy tales. New York: Vintage Books.

Nowlin C. (1929). The story teller and his pack (pp. 267-288). Springfield, MA: Milton Bradley Co.

# NEWSLETTER

## Definition

*Newsletter* is a publication of a collection of articles, anecdotes, and/or letters mailed to many people.

## Purposes

- Shares information among persons with similar interests, goals, and activities.
- Educates readers and keeps them in touch by sending announcements, reports, or information needed to take action.
- Communicates personally with many people and promotes an idea or activity.
- Entertains readers -- for some groups, an appropriate goal.

---

**Advantages**

- The newsletter is a relatively inexpensive way to convey information to many people.
- It can be prepared quickly.
- It can be addressed to a group with specialized interests.
- It can provide a means of continuing education in a variety of subjects.
- Because newsletters are usually chatty, informal, and personal, they are likely to hold a reader's interest.

**Disadvantages**

- Newsletters can be used too often, and thus lose interest and impact.
- Mailing lists need constant revision.
- A good newsletter can take a lot of work; it should not be assumed to be an easy form of communication that can be prepared casually or hurriedly.

---

## Preparation of the Newsletter

- In deciding to start or continue publishing a newsletter, determine whether another, more effective way is available to get the information across.
- Decisions must be made about finances and distribution, as well as publication or preparation.
- Mechanical considerations.
  a. You need attention catchers, such as appropriate illustrations.
  b. Printing must be uniform and appealing.
  c. Duplication must be done well.
  d. Text must be well spaced and centered on page.
  e. Avoid spelling errors, use of incorrect grammar, and improper punctuation.
  f. Seek assistance from persons knowledgeable about editing and designing a newsletter.

## Points to Remember

- Timing of mailings is important.
- Readers' reactions to form and content should be encouraged and utilized.
- The impact of the newsletter needs periodic evaluation.

## References

Cooper, S. (1983). Methods of teaching revisited, newsletters and pamphlets. Journal of Continuing Education in Nursing, 14, 25-27.

Cooper, S. (1988). Teaching tips: The periodically printed word: An alternative teaching method. Journal of Continuing Education in Nursing, 19 (1), 43-44.

Morgan, B., Holmes, G., & Bundy. (1976). Methods in adult education (34th ed.). Danville, IL: Interstate Printers and Publishers. (A brief discussion of newsletters for adults.)

Wales, L. (1976). A practical guide to newsletter editing and design Ames, IA: Iowa State University Press. (A "how-to" book that gives instructions and ideas for various aspects of newsletter editing and design. Available from Iowa State University Press, South State Avenue, Ames, IA 50010.)

# NEWSPAPER

## Definition

*Newspaper* is a publication regularly printed and distributed; (usually daily or weekly) containing news, opinions, advertisements and other items of general interest.

## Purposes

- A living textbook that spans the textbook lag.
- Study and analyze current events.
- Observe historical trends, since it is a chronicle of history.
- May be used to teach skills of critical reviewing.
- Increase verbal participation of learners.
- May be used to provide medium for written materials.

---

**Advantages**

- Provides local, national and international perspective.
- May be used by individuals or groups, for many disciplines, and to teach many skills.
- May be combined with displays or collections.
- Useful for any age of reader to motivate learning and desire to read.
- Flexible for a wide variety of information, topics, and subjects.
- May be reproduced and or projected (overhead transparencies, opaque projector).
- Readily available and inexpensive.

**Disadvantages**

- Quality of reporting and writing varies.
- May not be viewed as a valuable educational tool.
- Print may be considered as "truth" and de-emphasize the "propaganda" aspect.

---

## Points to Remember

- Need to plan for its use with instructions and activities.
- Learning through reading the paper:
  a. Learners need guidance as to the who, what, when, why and how of news stories.
  b. Purpose for reading should be clear -- is detail needed or will skimming suffice?
- Learning through writing the paper:
  a. Learners may need suggestions, direction, and/or assistance.
  b. See creative tool used by one nurse who wrote a weekly column about family health care (Staab).

**Suggestions for Preserving Old Clippings Forever**

Mix two teaspoons of magnesium carbonate and a quart of club soda in a large plastic dish. Sandwich the clippings between two pieces of screen of Pellon (a material sold in fabric stores) and soak for 30 minutes. Mop up excess water with blotting paper and allow to dry overnight on more blotting paper. Store clipping in well-sealed flat plastic bag. (National Archives)

**References**

Brown, J. W., et al. (1969). AV instruction -- materials and methods (3rd ed.). New York: McGraw-Hill.

Cooper, S. S. (1983). A potpourri of teaching techniques. Journal of Continuing Education in Nursing, 14(1), 3639.

Gustafson, M. (1986). Teaching tips: Advice columns as a teaching tool. Journal of Continuing Education in Nursing, 16(5), 181.

Heitzman, W. R. (1979). The newspaper in the classroom. Washington, DC: National Education Association.

Landers, A. (1968). Ann Landers says truth is stranger. Englewood Cliffs, NJ: Prentice Hall, Inc.

Stabb, A. (1978, November 30). Nurse's tools for teaching a newspaper. The American Nurse, 10(10),9.
(American Newspaper Publishers Association Foundation. P.O. Box 17407, Dulles International Airport, Washington, DC, 20041.) (This source of information on using the newspaper in teaching will also be helpful in identifying a newspaper educator in your region).

# NURSING ROUNDS

**Definition**

*Nursing Rounds* is when a small group of nurses come together to discuss nursing care.

**Purposes**

- Develop all facets of nursing process.
- Develop communication skills.
- Expand and reinforce theoretical content.
- Share nursing care plans.
- Introduce new or unfamiliar equipment and procedures.
- Develop peer review skills.
- Compare patient experiences and nursing care.

---

**Advantages**

- Way to promote peer assistance and peer review.
- Instructors can serve as role models.
- Way to provide early exposure to clinical experience.
- Learners can develop the skills of orally describing their plan of care.
- Patient care improved as a result of group communication -- e.g., more consistency.

**Disadvantages**

- May interrupt the schedules for staff and/or patient care delivery.

---

**Format**

- Introduction
  acquaint learners with the purpose of the rounds.
- Discussion
  allow time for all to share and discussion to occur.
- Evaluation discussion
  summarize learning.

**Modifications**

- The rounds may be conducted by the instructor, a learner, a group of learners, or a staff member.
- The patient and family may be included in the nursing round to get their perspective on care.

**Points to Remember**

- Schedule a time that is convenient for the staff, and learners, if possible.
- Prepare the learners for the experience.
- Readings may be recommended to learners prior to the rounds.
- Introduce all participants.
- Actively involve everyone in the discussion.
- Limit the group to 5-6 learners.
- Limit the time to 15-20 minutes.

**References**


Malasanos, L. (1977). The bedside clinic -- Nursing rounds as a teaching strategy. Journal of Nursing Education, 16 (6), 10-15.

Schweer, J., & Gabbie, K. (1976). Creative teaching in clinical nursing (3rd ed., pp. 120-121). St. Louis: C.V. Mosby.

Smith, L., & Hudson, M. (1984). Physical assessment rounds as a teaching strategy. Journal of Nursing Education, 23 30-32.

# OBJECT

## Definition

*Objects* are real things which have been removed from natural setting.

## Purpose

- Bridge gap between known and unknown.
- Acquaint with reality.
- Clarify concepts.
- Permit an accurate impression.
- Attract attention.
- Make learning uniform -- all see the same thing.

---

## Advantages

- Increase educational value.
- Readily available and generally familiar.
- May appeal to several senses -- touch, sight, smell, taste.
- Detail can be appreciated.
- Inexpensive.
- Avoid going on tour by bringing object to class.
- Supplement verbal information.
- Unfamiliar may hold interest -- promotes curiosity.
- May be used in combination -- display, exhibit.

## Disadvantages

- Some real things may be:
  - too large to be convenient, may be too awkward to use.
  - too small to see or handle.
  - too delicate or transient to handle or keep.
  - too complex to understand.
  - too difficult to find nearby.
  - too dangerous.
  - too removed from natural site to have meaning.
  - too expensive for multiple usage.

---

## Source of Objects

- Teacher may collect, prepare, purchase.
- Students may collect and contribute.
- Teacher may wish to keep a file of sources.

## Points to Remember

- Be sure all can see.
- If possible, pass object and allow for touch.
- Do not talk while object is circulating.
- May wish to link solid object with picture (enlarged).
- May be helpful to show picture of object in natural surroundings.

**Other Related Methodologies:** Object Lesson, Specimens.

## References

Brown, J. W., Lewis, R. B., & Harcleroad, F. (1964). A-V Instruction materials and methods (2nd ed.). New York: McGraw-Hill.

Saunders, D. J. (1979). Visual communication handbook. London: United Society for Christian Literature.

# OBJECT LESSON

## Definition

*Object Lesson* is a teaching method using an object with a story.

## Purpose

- Draw parallel of physical qualities of object with a story, parable, or allegory.
- Teach concepts.

---

**Advantages**

- Inexpensive.
- Connect familiar object with a concept.
- Use objects and illustrations drawn from everyday life.
- Young and old find interesting and fascinating.

**Disadvantages**

- If the meaning is missed, it is entertainment, not learning.
- Younger children not capable of understanding symbolic meaning.
- If mystery and trickery involved, may be associated with supernatural.
- Mysterious element may detract from main concept.

---

## Points to Remember

- Practice and become familiar with objects/parts/equipment.
- Be sure object is large enough and all can see.
- Keep all objects together in one box and conceal them until they are used.
- Draw parallels that are genuine and not strained.
- Do not overdo it. Two or three good points are better than six or seven exaggerated ones.
- Avoid gadgets or very complicated parts if they detract from the central concepts.
- Correlate length of lesson with attention span of learners.
- Correlate object in view with significant points.
- You may wish to summarize and reinforce the learning.
- It may be appropriate to have learners tell what they learned, to check for understanding.
- Teacher may wish to keep a file of ready-made lessons, ideas, objects, or sources.

**Other Related Methodologies:** Objects, Magic, Storytelling.

## References


Getz, G. A. (1972). Audiovisual media. Chicago: Moody Press.

➢ Saunders, D. J. (1979). Visual communication handbook. London: United Society for Christian Literature.

# OBSERVATION

## Definition

*Observation* (planned) is the act or practice of noting and recording facts or events, for scientific study or performance evaluation.

## Purposes

- Note specific actions, activities and procedures to be studied.
- Increase awareness of many facts of a situation.
- Influence and change attitudes and insights.
- Increase abilities of data gathering.
- Provide feedback to daily performance.

---

**Advantages**

- Can provide unified experiences for a group.
- May be used with many other methods -- demonstration, study tour etc.
- Expedient, may save time for learners.
- Provides more time to see the "whole" than when learner is the doer.

**Disadvantages**

- Requires careful planning and several stages.
- Activities may become random and purposeless.
- Learner may desire to be a doer rather than an observer.
- Teacher is less able to control some settings.

---

## Points to Remember

- Learners may need to develop curiosity and effective habits of observation.
- Learner needs to know what to observe for and what he/she is (and is not) responsible for.
- Teacher needs to plan step by step, include time for discussion, reporting, and sharing.
- Teacher may wish to provide written instructions of other structured forms.
- For additional information on observer role, see guideline for multiple assignment.

**Other Related Methodologies:** Demonstration, Study Tour, Exhibit, Films, Videos, Multiple Student Assignment.

## References


Dale, E. (1976). Audio-visual methods in teaching (3rd ed.). New York: Dryden Press.

Schulman, J., Foley, J., & Voorsanger, E. (1966). Observation of a hospitalized child as a teacher technique in a student nurse's education. Journal of Nursing Education, 5(4), 7-12.

## OPAQUE PROJECTION

**Definition**

*Opaque Projection* is the projection of opaque material (through which no light can pass) by means of reflected light.

**Purposes**

- Projects materials without any special preparation.
- Shows samples of student's work
- Displays pictures on paper or board.
- Enlarges or makes large-scale drawing or maps for other uses (poster, scenery).
- Projects in silhouette (coins, shells, tools, fabrics, plants).

---

**Advantages**

- It is unnecessary to process projection materials.
- Any book or picture can be projected instantly and in color, without any special preparation.
- The method is useful when you have only one copy of materials.
- There is no need to remove a page from a book.
- In a small group, opaque projection can show much detail.
- Small, flat equipment can be demonstrated.
- Cost of equipment is not prohibitive (screen can be used with other projectors).
- Equipment is simple to set up and operate.
- An image can be kept on screen as long as required.
- Everyone sees the same thing at the same time.

**Disadvantages**

- Opaque projection requires a darkened room.
- It requires functioning electrical equipment -- projector and screen.
- Large classes may not see as much detail.
- It may be distracting if teacher uses material with print too small to be read.
- Projector is large and somewhat cumbersome.
- Materials left in machine (especially an old one) may be damaged by overheating.

---

**Points to Remember**

- Any familiar situation can be illustrated pictorially.
- You may project almost anything -- pictures, postcards, photographs.
- Projections may be supplemented with handouts, tape recordings.

- Use where copyright laws restrict copying of printed materials.
- Check equipment prior to class; it may be wise to have a spare bulb on hand.
- Test clarity of projection on screen for size and distortion.
- Practice using equipment. Read instructions.

**References**


Dale, E. (1976). Audiovisual methods in teaching (3rd ed., pp. 457-458). New York: Dryden Press, Holt, Rinehart and Winston.

Kinder, J. (1973). Using instructional media (pp. 75-76). New York: D. Van Nostrand.

# OVERHEAD PROJECTOR

## Definition

*Overhead Projector* is an electrical device designed to project transparent material as large as 10" x 10" and as small as 2" x 2".

## Purposes

- Provide visual material to support a speaker presentation.
- Increase retention.
- Maximize interest.
- Show relationships.
- Explain material -- such as with charts, maps, diagrams.
- Encourage participation -- as with discussion and initiating brainstorming.
- Substitute for a chalkboard or flip chart.

---

## Advantages

- Versatile -- may be used by any teacher, for almost any age, in any audience, any auditorium, to teach any subject.
- Allows for maximum creativity.
- Simple -- no special operator is necessary; easy to use.
- Convenient -- the projected image is visible in a lighted room, projector is light weight (some portables are lighter than others), overhead transparencies make note taking easy, class time can be saved by having similar or identical material prepared in advance, a screen may not be necessary.
- Effective -- projector is used in front of the class, teacher can face the class, the projected image is always in full view of the instructor as he faces the class, ideas can be presented one at a time, emphasis may be obtained by underlining words, adding color, or using a pointer, there are several interesting and effective techniques that can be achieved, conclusions of a discussion can be summarized at once.
- Economical -- transparencies may be made inexpensively, transparencies may be used repeatedly and stored easily.

## Disadvantages

- An electrical machine requires electricity, a handy outlet, and a bulb that works.
- Projector and screen may have to be transported from place to place.
- Time is required to creatively develop good transparencies.
- Requires facility to talk and use transparency simultaneously.
- Careless teachers may utilize it improperly or overuse the tool.

---

## **Methods Used in Making Transparencies**

- Impromptu (in class): Writing or drawing on single sheets or rolls.
- Handmade (prior to class): Writing or drawing with special pens, applying transfers, typewriting or pasting cutouts on transparencies.
- Machine-processed: By spirit duplicator, thermal copy, diazo (ammonia process), lift or picture transfer, electrostatic film, or by photocopy film.
- Commercially produced: Finished transparencies and overlays, from paper masters.

## **Equipment Needed**

- Basic or "must" haves include:
  Transparency Markers
  (1) Pencils -- although grease pencils are the cheapest, they are not as satisfactory.
  (2) Pens -- Felt tip pens in a variety of colors. These should state they are for use on transparencies. Not all will work equally well.
    (a) Water soluble -- non permanent that may be removed with water.
    (b) Permanent -- may be removed with rubbing alcohol without marring the material.
  Transparent Plastic
  (1) X-ray film is the cheapest but may require cleaning. May be cleaned by thoroughly washing off exposed film with full strength household bleach. Follow caution in use of rubber gloves, plastic apron, not splashing in eyes, and using well ventilated area. Rinse with clear water and hang up to dry.
  (2) Acetate in sheets or rolls. Substitute may be clear sheets from photo albums, and report covers.
  (3) Polyester Sheets -- the most satisfactory and durable material because it has plasticizer in it, which keeps it from getting brittle with age. Five mil (.005) is thick enough for average use.
- Additional useful helps:
  Grid sheets
  Gadget box
  (1) Contains such items as scissors, compass, clear plastic protractor, single edged razor. You may wish to purchase a starter set which will contain pens and some of these items.
  Pattern file (may contain figures and/or comic strips).

## **Suggestions for Making Maximum-Impact Transparencies**

- Visibility:
  1. Maximize image size. Failure to do this is probably the number one cause for disinterest
  2. Use the horizontal format.
  3. Lettering should be no less than 1/4 inch high. Generally, use capital letters. Formula: Size letter x .8 x distance projected in feet equals size of image. Example: 1/4" letter x .8 x 12 feet equals 2.4 inch letters on screen.
  4. Fonts of 24 points or greater size are the best.

- Clarity
  1. Minimize the content -- failure to do this is probably the number two cause of disinterest.
  2. Concentrate one point or one comparison per visual.
  3. Use step by step procedure in breaking down complex idea or subject.
- Simplicity
  1. Normally one idea per transparency.
  2. 6-8 words maximum per line.
  3. 8-10 lines maximum per visual.
- Use of color
  1. Blue is the best all around color for printing.
  2. Vivid, intense colors are especially important when the room is fully lighted.
  3. Use color in illustrations and objects as well as printing.
  4. Decorations may add, provided they do not clutter.
- Use of variety
  1. Use illustrations.
  2. Use overlays, masks, graphics, adhesive colored acetate, and dry transfer letters for the professional look.
  3. Photos can also be transferred onto transparencies at your local copy center.

**Using Machine-Processed**

- Thermofax or Heat Process Machine
  1. Follow instructions with the machine on settings and directions.
  2. The secret to good transparencies with these machines is the use of carbon in the original.
  3. Large solid areas will not reproduce well.
  4. Xerox copies, newspapers, black and white magazine pages, and mimeograph work; all contain enough carbon to reproduce with this process.
  5. Colors, ditto paper, ball-point pens and felt-tip pens will not reproduce.
  6. Make your original on white paper, but not erasable bond paper.
  7. Use a backing sheet if you use a small item, such as a newspaper clipping.
- Con-Tact Lifting or making a transparency from a clay-coated magazine. Since this is quite detailed, it is suggested you find this described elsewhere -- such as in the reference by Noren.
- Diazo Process involves a chemical process and directions may be found in some audio-visual books that discuss inexpensive methods. The reference by Noren is one such source.

**Using Transparencies Effectively**

- Stage and lamp must be clean, check functioning before presentation.
- Position projector properly, with screen in the center or corner of the room.
- For maximum visibility, the image should be projected as high in the room as possible.
- Check the size of print, adjust for best viewing.
- Keep the lights on, dim if appropriate.
- Organize transparencies in order to be shown.
- Consider overlays to simplify the complex.

- Use a pointer or pencil. If your hand is "shaky", place it rather than hold it.
- Underline important points.
- Use flat objects as silhouettes.
- Check focus during presentation. But do not keep looking at the screen or speaking to it.
- Turn off lamp during gaps in transparency presentation. Do not leave it on to distract attention when not needed.
- Distribute handouts at best time in relationship to viewing and note taking.
- Include the usefulness of transparencies as a part of the presentation evaluation questions.

**Mounting and Storing**

- Frame or mount heavily used transparencies with cardboard or paper.
- It is generally easier to use mounted transparencies than unmounted.
- There is less damage to the transparency if mounted and stored with paper between each.
- Writing notes on or attaching to the frame is neater and conveys preparedness and organization.
- A well organized system is essential for reuse. Folders or notebook may be used.

**References**


Bauman, K., & Kirkman, A. (1979). Overhead transparencies: The overlooked medium. Nurse Educator, 4(4), 21-25. (Nine steps, use and misuse are discussed.)

Clark, C. (1988). Transparencies: let them work for you. Nurse Educator, 13(2), 21-22.

Darkes, A. S. (1977). How to make and use overhead transparencies. Chicago: Moody Press. (Intended as a very complete guide for religious education workers who wish to make inexpensive transparencies and use them effectively.)

Kinder, J. S. Using instructional media (pp. 76-79). New York: D. Van Nostrand Co. (Basic information on the use of the overhead projector.)

Lange, C. M. (1976). Using the overhead projector. Nursing Outlook, 24(3), 145.

Morgan, B., Holmes, G. F., & Bundy, D. E. (1976). Methods in adult education (3rd ed.). Danville, IL: The Interstate Printers & Publishers, Inc. (Excellent source on the use of this method in adult education.)

Noren, C. (1976). Teaching over my head. Creative use of the overhead project. Elgin, IL: David C. Cook Publishing Co. (A very practical step-by-step book intended for those working in religious education and having limited funds to purchase commercial materials.)

Pettibone, T. J. (1976). Overhead transparency legibility as a function of distance image reversal and letter height and width. Audio-Visual Journal, 11(1), 84-88. (Report on a research study related to aspects listed in the title of the article.)

# PAMPHLET

## Definition

*Pamphlet* is a booklet of printed matter.

## Purposes

- Provide concise, easy to read information.
- Influences attitudes and behavior.
- Informs and motivates.
- Supplements usual source material.

---

**Advantages**

- Pamphlets are available from numerous official and private agencies.
- They are inexpensive or free.
- Each student may have his/her own copy.

**Disadvantages**

- Pamphlets are often misused or discarded without being read.
- They must be used in conjunction with other methods.
- They need to be reviewed by the teacher.
- Time is required to prepare one's own.

---

## Checklist for Evaluation of Pamphlets

- ✓ Are the scientific facts accurate?
- ✓ Is the information pertinent?
- ✓ Is it presented clearly?
- ✓ Do selection and arrangement constitute good coverage?
- ✓ Are the ideas significant?
- ✓ Is it worth the time to prepare, preview, and use in this course?
- ✓ Is the content free of unsound or untrue claims?
- ✓ Does it have interest appeal?
- ✓ Is there a mixture of familiar and new material to foster growth?
- ✓ Is the degree of motivation of action sufficiently potent?

## Points to Remember

- ➢ A pamphlet needs to be simple.
- ➢ It must have a definite message.
- ➢ It is important to use bold print, lots of color, illustrations, and ample white space.
- ➢ A pamphlet must be appropriate to the age and reading level of the audience.

- Good paper stock should be used to provide color, contrast, and lack of glare.
- Typography, design, and illustration should be attractive and effective.
- The value of a pamphlet depends on how and when it is used.

## References

Brown, J., et al. (1959). A-V instruction materials and methods (pp. 70-95). New York: McGraw-Hill. (A chapter on free and inexpensive materials, sources of pamphlets, and how to obtain them.)

Morgan, B., Holmes, G., & Bundy, C. (1976). Methods in adult education (3rd ed.). Danville, IL: Interstate Printers and Publishers. (Contains a brief section on bulletins, leaflets, circulars, and pamphlets.)

# PANEL

## Definition

*Panel* is an experience in group discussion where a group of experts under the guidance of a leader or moderator, share information and ideas with a larger audience. Usually involves 5-8 experts.

Panel members present their materials in an informal, conversational manner (as opposed to a symposium, where members read prepared papers). (Wandelt).

A presentation in which a small group discusses a topic or issue without making prepared speeches. Either with or without active participation by the audience. (Good)

## Purposes

- To provide a volume of information in a short time.
- To present different aspects of a complicated subject.
- To present different points of view.
- To present an area in which listeners have insufficient knowledge or the knowledge area is too large for discussion.
- To present a topic in which no one individual can present the entire subject.

---

**Advantages**

- Can take less time than a lecture to present more information.
- Exposure to highly specialized experience of experts and various points of view.
- Retain interest by use of a variety of speakers.

**Disadvantages**

- Conflicting points of view may confuse audience.
- Inadequate preparation for panel participation may lead to lack of cohesiveness and goal direction. (Possible disadvantages of having a guest speaker multiplied).

---

## How to Use

- Select subject matter which builds on listener's prior knowledge.
- Present all points of view.
- Panel members introduce topic and set tone, and then audience enters discussion.
- Accommodations.
  a. Panel members should be seated in semicircle or V-shaped arrangement.
  b. Moderator sits in middle.

- Rules for all members (Wandelt).
  a. Each member assumes responsibility for helping all other members tell their stories.
  b. Each member keeps the central theme in mind and assumes responsibility for keeping the group on the topic and from moving the discussion forward.
  c. Each member has a 3 minute time limit at any one time.
  d. Each member follows the discussion and keeps it on a conversational plane by interjecting questions and comments.
- Roles of Participants.
  a. Moderator or leader
     1) Introduce topic and panel members.
     2) Outline procedure and how audience will participate.
     3) Guide and control discussion -- among members and with audience.
     4) Try to equalize participation and get all points of view presented.
     5) Summarize discussion.
  b. Panel members
     1) Need not be <u>the</u> experts on the subject but at least as well informed as the majority of expected audience.
     2) Use authoritative resources of own expertise to substantiate information or point of view.
     3) Promote equal participation -- not dominate.
- Preparation for Panel Participation.
  a. Select members for knowledge of subject and skill in presentation.
  b. Invite Panelists to participate.
     1) clearly define topic.
     2) clearly identify particular facet on which panelist will speak.
  c. If possible meet with panelist (or communicate by letter) to:
     1) meet other participants.
     2) outline discussion.
     3) assign responsibilities.
     4) reinforce fact that presentation is informal.
  d. Meet shortly before presentation to:
     1) recheck outline.
     2) work out time allocation.
     3) set mood for cooperative participation.

**References**

Bormann, E. (1969). Discussion and group methods: Theory & practice (pp. 34-35). New York: Harper and Row. (Brief description of a panel with some practical suggestions for planning that can create the illusion of a spontaneous, informal conference.)

Cooper, S. (1979). Methods of teaching-revisited. Panel discussion. Journal of Continuing Education in Nursing, 10(2), 36-38.

Ford, L. (1970). Using the panel in teaching and training. Nashville: TN: Boardmann Press. (A cartoon book giving basic principles of the use of the panel. Useful sketches.)

Good, C. V. (1959). Dictionary of education (2nd ed.). New York: McGraw-Hill.

Moran, E. (1953). Panels don't have to be dull. American Journal of Nursing, 53, 571-572.

Wandelt, M. (1959). Vital panel. American Journal of Nursing, 59(5), 672-675. (Outlines the careful preparation necessary for a successful panel discussion. Presents the four basic rules for panel members. Helpful article.)

# PANTOGRAPH

## Definition

*Pantograph* is a device for mechanical duplication of drawings or designs in enlarged or reduced scale

## Purposes

- Enlarge or reduce original drawings, designs, pictures, and other materials.
- Permit change in size of object without damage to original.
- Useful tool in preparing visual materials for various projected and non-projected media.

---

**Advantages**

- Inexpensive.
- Readily available (art supply, toy store).
- Requires no prior experience.
- No danger to original.

**Disadvantages**

- May require some manipulation to determine enlargement or reduction.
- Lack of or unclear instructions may result in increased time to determine operation.

---

## Equipment Required

- Pantograph
- Table or hard surface that will not be damaged.
- Original drawing, design, or picture to be enlarged or reduced.
- Drawing pins or tape.
- Paper for the reproduced drawing.
- Pencil.

## Points to Remember

- As the marking pin is moved along the outline of the original drawing, the drawing pencil will reproduce the sketch in the desired size, depending on the adjustment on the drawing paper.
- The larger the number selected, the larger the enlargement.
- Screws must be placed on the same number.
- The eye should be focused on the marking pin at all times.

# PARABLE

## Definition

*Parable* is a short, simple, direct narrative that teaches a truth by means of a fictitious examples.

## Purposes

- To tell a story in an ancient form of storytelling.
- Teach a higher order moral or religious truth.
- Incorporate contemporary principles with traditional beliefs and values.

---

## Advantages

- Is common form of storytelling to many accustomed to the oral tradition.
- Easy to use -- need only imagination.
- Short and simple, may be either direct or indirect.
- May be extemporaneous or planned, may be borrowed and modified.
- Appropriate to all ages.
- A subtle way to suggest problem solving of problems in a culturally acceptable manner.
- Acknowledges local, traditional beliefs and values.
- May be combined with visualizations (A-V aids, drama) or music (may be sung).

## Disadvantages

- Requires knowledge of local culture for maximum effectiveness.
- In retelling and repetition, the main objective may be lost.
- In non-literate societies, known for entertainment value.

---

## Points to Remember

- Body and spirit of the parables -- the narrative and its interpretation are kept separate
- Scenario is lifted from local culture (names, locations, customs).
- Base it on educational objective.
- Keep it short and simple.
- Must be told, not read.

## Examples/Sources

- May be difficult to find. Some from India and Greece. Most common are found in Holy Bible.
- Health education examples are beginning to be available.

**Other Related Methodologies:** Allegory, Fable, Folk tale

**References**

Hilton, D. (1978, July). Teaching through storytelling. Salubritas, 2(3), 4-5. (An exciting example of the use of parables, including a parable, from a physician in northeastern Nigeria.)

Werner, D., & Bower, B. (1986). Helping health workers learn. Palo Alto, CA: Hesperian Foundation.

# PEER REVIEW

## Definition

*Peer Review* is objective validation of the performance of a peer.

## Purposes

- A method of evaluating and improving practice or teaching.
- May be used to identify group (or department) needs for further learning, such as a workshop.
- A method which may be used in selection and/or retention.
- A measure of accountability.
- Provides opportunity for developing skill in giving and receiving feedback.

## Rationale

- Increasing importance is being given to peer review as a professional function of educators.

- Provides the learner with assistance from peers, as well as preceptors and educators which should be valuable in preparation for future responsibility.

## Responsibilities When Using Peer Review

- Since psychological threat is involved in evaluation, mutual trust needs to be developed.
- The reviewee and reviewer need to establish a mutual contract for the review; spelling out objectives, approach and criteria to be used.
- The one being reviewed makes the final decisions in implementation of plans.
- Peer review should be a continuing, ongoing, up-to-date process rather than an annual review or something quickly enacted.
- Criteria may be developed by a group or panel and mutually agreed upon.
- Research on peer review should be planned and incorporated for institutions and groups intending to use the method.

## Other Related Uses

May be combined very effectively with videotaping or observation.

## References

Burnside, I. M. (1971). Peer supervision: A method of teaching. Journal of Nursing Education, 10(3), 15-22. (Faculty member describes experiences with eight students, working in pairs during a quarter of master's program in psychiatric nursing.)

Gorecki, Y. (1977). Faculty peer review. Nursing Outlook, 25(7), 439-442. (Faculty in a diploma program describe their experiences.)

Gold, H., Jackson, J., Sachs, B., & Van Meter, M. (1973). Peer review--A working experiment. Nursing Outlook, 21(10), 634-636. (The report of an experiment at the University of Michigan, University hospitals.)

Hauser, M. A. (1975). Initiation into peer review. American Journal of Nursing, 75(12), 2204-2207. (A brief account of peer review experienced by a nurse at a Veteran's home.)

Hinshaw, A. S., & Field, M. A. (1974). An investigation of variables that underline collegial evaluation. Nursing Research, 23(4), 292-300. (A study by two nurse scientists in Sociology at University of Arizona, using Blau's theory and studying professional nursing staff at University hospitals.)

Johnson, K., & Zimmerman, M. A. Peer review in health department. American Journal of Nursing, 75(4), 618-619. (A brief article describing the annual evaluation in a county community health facility.)

Page, S., & Loeper, J. (1978). Peer review of the nurse educator, the process and the development of a format. Journal of Nursing Education, 17(9), 21-29. (Two graduate students report the findings of their study of faculty peer review.)

# PHILATELY

## Definition

*Philately* is the collection and study of postage stamps and stationary marked with postal cancellations. Synonymous with stamp collecting.

## Purposes

- Creates interest in a common item that may give historical perspective.
- Fosters inquiry and investigation.
- Provides an international perspective to issues.

---

**Advantages**

- Many stamps are readily available and inexpensive.
- Stamps are unique and interesting.
- Philately builds on information and interest some learners may already possess.
- Stamps portray in an authentic way historical and current emphasis on various issues.
- Stamps are a creative teaching tool that is widely overlooked.

**Disadvantages**

- Some stamps and information about them may be difficult to obtain.
- Hobby may become expensive.

---

## Points to Remember

- Stimulate interest in trends, individuals, and international issues.
- Correlate societal actions with occurrences within the nursing profession (stamps honoring various persons and agencies).
- Stamps may be used singly to introduce a topic, draw out a learner with specific interest, or in a display or collection.
- There are collections available for rent, as well as slide collections. (See RN Magazine pamphlet listed below.)

## References


Brown, J. W., et al. (1969). Audio-visual instruction, media and methods (pp. 374-376). New York: McGraw-Hill.

Daniloff, R. (1976). Getting into the stamp act. American Education, 12(1), 16-22. (Suggests uses of stamps as interest-catching classroom aids that touch just about every conceivable subject.)

Diffenbaugh, D. J. (1975). Fun with stamps in environmental studies. Science Teacher, 42(5), 57-58.

Florence Nightingale. Postage stamp celebrating 150th anniversary issued by Great Britain. American Journal of Nursing, 70(5), 953.

From your stamp album. (1973). Iceland's nursing stamp is issued. (news item). American Journal of Nursing, 73(11), 1973.

Hamilton, M. C. (1975). Stamp history into their minds. Instructor, 85(2), 104-106.

RN Magazine's Collection of Stamps Honoring Nursing. (1970). Oradell, NJ: Medical Economics, Co.

Slesnick, I., & Whitmer, J. (1976). Phenomena for inquiry? Postage stamps. Science and Children, 40(1), 40.

# PICTIONARY

## Definition

*Pictionary* is a board game or charades on paper, introduced in 1986.

## Purposes

- Take advantage of the nation's most popular game (Pictionary is #1, Monopoly is #4).
- Modify a known game for specific educational content.
- Plan for learning to be fun.

---

**Advantages**

- A game considered acceptable as adult activity.
- Any age can play.
- Forces interaction and socialization.
- Is a noncompetitive game.
- Can be prepared by the teacher or students.
- Allows for cross-cultural interaction even with language limitations.

**Disadvantages**

- May be seen as entertainment and less than educational.
- Is connected to noncompetitive, "mindless" fun.
- Some time is required to prepare the "ideas" to be drawn.
- Some familiarity with the commercial game is necessary to modify the game.

---

## References

Gustafson, M. (1991). Board games with a health focus. Health World, 2 (8), 13-14.

Rix, H. (1998, February 5). Pictionary is charades on paper. The Minneapolis Star Tribune, p. 3E.

William, L. (1989, November 5). Adults play more -- in noncompetitive games. The Minneapolis Star Tribune, p. 1E.

# POLAR MOTION

## Definition

*Polar Motion* is a technique to convey concepts of motion on overhead transparencies, slides and other visuals. Motion is achieved through variable oriented polarized light.

## Purpose

- Simulate realistic motion.
- Convey concepts of sequence, flow, and cause and effect.
- Create unusual effects on and off, turbulence, swirling, rotating, flow and radiation.

---

**Advantages**

- Adds interest through motion.

**Disadvantages**

- Requires one more piece of equipment (hand operated or manual or motor driven polarized filter or spinner).
- Requires special stressed plastic be applied to areas of transparency and used with spinner.
- Additional cost of materials and equipment.*

---

* (The price [in 1979] of one mechanical model was about $50.00 and the hand operated filter very inexpensive.)

## Points to Remember

- Follow instructions on materials for placement.
- Be sure special plastic is correctly placed to insure correct direction of motion or action.

**Other Related Methodologies:** Polarizing, Technamation.

## References


Kemp, J. (1975). Planning and producing audiovisual materials(3rd ed., pp. 198, 216, 304). New York: Thomas Crowell. (Lists sources of materials and equipment.)

Minor, E. (1978). Handbook for preparing visual media (2nd ed., pp. 218-219). New York: McGraw-Hill. (Gives instructions on using materials and the spinner.)

## POLAROID

**Definition**

*Polaroid* is a commercial camera that allows for "instant" photography.

**Purpose**

- Take prints and slides that can immediately be used.
- Capitalize on a source of providing teaching photographs.

---

**Advantages**

- Available for prints and slides, in color and black and white.
- Prints are made and may be used immediately.
- No need for a darkroom or other equipment.
- Relatively inexpensive.
- Students may use in class.

**Disadvantages**

- Equipment requires some understanding to achieve good results.
- If class is large and individual or small groups need duplicates of cameras, may become expensive.

---

**Points to Remember**

- Very effective with photograph learners.
- Use for bulletin board materials.
- Use to make prints for story board in preparing other visuals.
- May be used to make Polaroid land projection transparencies for which a lantern slide projector is needed. (Homemade transparency from Polaroid is also possible-see article by Williams.)

**Other Related Methodologies:** Photographs (Snapshot), Photostory.

**References**


Minor, E. (1978). Handbook for preparing visual media (2nd ed., p. 158). New York: McGraw-Hill. (briefly discusses uses.)

Williams, B. (1974). Projecting Polaroid photographs. Science Teacher, 41. (Explains use by students.)

# POSTCARD

## Definition

*Postcard* is a card bearing a message and/or picture through the mails without an envelope.

## Purposes

- An innovative teaching tool made by placing a specific illustration on a card.
- Arouse curiosity in a subject, topic, or object by sending a picture via the public mails.

---

**Advantages**

- May be specific to a culture.
- Inexpensive
- Versatile, most places have some postal services.
- Simple to make.
- Creates awareness in a natural way.
- Stimulates interest, curiosity, and discussion among receivers/readers.
- May be used in combination with literacy classes.

**Disadvantages**

- May be dependent on delivery time, and thus take some flexibility in planning.
- Illustrations on teaching postcards must be well planned.
- Could be overused and lose effectiveness, novelty, and fun.

---

## Points to Remember

- Keep illustration and/or instructions simple.
- Select appropriate individual to receive card.
- May be wise to test how long it took to arrive and who read the card.
- May send in a series or collect in a book for serial effect.
- If combined with literacy classes, plan follow-up and check to see what was understood.

## References

Tisa, B. (1984, Spring-Summer). A village mailman's story -- The potential of postcards. Appropriate Technology for Health (pp. 14-15). Newsletter. Geneva, Switzerland: WHO (p. 25).

Tisa, B. (1980, January). The village mailman: The potential of postcards. Development Communication Report (pp. 14-15). Washington, DC: AID, #29.

# POSTER

## Definition

*Poster* is a placard, based on one dominant, simplified idea; for posting.

## Purposes

- Persuades the reader to take action based on the facts presented.
- Communicates a significant idea quickly.
- Announces events, promote campaigns or issues.
- Stimulates interest and curiosity, attracts attention.
- Gathers ideas and insights of learners.

---

## Advantages

- Posters exert great visual power.
- They may be specifically made or purchased to meet an objective or event.
- They are inexpensive.
- They are useful for almost any age group.
- They can employ pictures and symbols for those with reading limitations.

## Disadvantages

- Symbolic nature may be misunderstood.
- A poster may be cluttered and unclear if it contains too many ideas, words, or pictures.
- It may be ignored if not carefully displayed and/or if on display too long.
- Posters may be overused.

---

## Suggestions for Preparation

- Communicate one idea.
- Limit number of words (five or fewer) and pictures or simple drawings.
- Be sure poster is large enough to be seen at intended distance.
- Use bold design, color, and lettering.
- Carefully plan for interest and good balance.
- Keep it fairly simple and uncluttered.
- Have equipment available if learners are to make their own (rulers, drawing pens, triangles).
- Lettering stencils, transfer letters, or computer graphics may give a more professional look.
- Interest may be added by use of a three-dimensional effect.
- It may be good to protect for permanent use with either clear plastic or a frame.
- The teacher may wish to collect and file posters.

## Points to Remember

- Place in a well-traveled area.
- Post in a variety of locations -- bulletin boards, kiosks, exhibits.
- Display at proper height with good lighting.
- Do not allow to get stagnant. Leave up no more than 2 weeks.
- It may be desirable to discuss poster in class.
- Learners may be involved in poster making through group preparation and/or a contest.
- Commercial or professional posters are available from a variety of sources, which range from free to very expensive (government agencies, public institutions, charitable organizations, groups such as the American Cancer Society).

**Other Related Methodologies:** Chart, Exhibit, Montage, Collage.

## References


Dale, E. (1969). Audiovisual methods in teaching (3rd ed., pp. 335-338). New York: Dryden Press, Holt, Rinehart and Winston. (Basic information about the use of posters in teaching.)

Donohue, B. (1978). Reusable print-cloth posters. Development Communication Report, 21, 6.

Kinder, J. (1973). Using instructional media (pp. 94-95). New York: D. Van Nostrand, Co.

Lange, C. (1976). Developing low-cost teaching materials. Nursing Outlook, 24(10), 614. (Posters and their use in nursing education.)

Melody, M., & Carrington, L. (1962). Poster explosion. American Journal of Nursing, 62(8), 92-93. (Handmade posters in in-service education.)

Preheim, L. (1988). Letters: Poster presenters' thumb. Medical Meetings, 15(6), 2.

**Definition**

*Poster Board Session* is a teaching system for presentation at a conference or convention.

**Purposes**

- Provide a more intimate forum for informal discussion.
- Provide an alternate form of presentation from that of giving oral papers.
- Utilize convention time effectively.
- Present information concisely.

---

**Advantages**

- Tailored to the needs of individual attendee.
- Allows direct exchange of ideas between author and participant(s) not possible during oral presentation.
- Provide for lively discussions.
- Allows more authors to share than could present papers.
- A low cost method of presentation for the conference planners.
- Presenters need not prepare a formal paper.

**Disadvantages**

- Committee may decide on this format when the presenter would prefer a traditional oral presentation.
- Not all material is conducive to the method.
- Requires careful planning and good visuals.
- Presenter may feel he is merely repeating basic information to a succession of attendees.
- Presenters generally are not paid.

---

**Points to Remember**

- Committee decides which papers will be presented in poster session.
- Instructions to presenters need to be very specific and clear.
- Presenters need to know basic rules and have instructions specific to the conference.

**Suggestions for Planners of Conference**

- You are responsible to solicit and determine who will present.
- Prepare specific written instructions. (May include diagram if standard format is desired.)
- Provide instructions well ahead so they can be used in preparing.

  How to prepare posters:

  1.) Size of board (____" long X ____" wide).

2.) Suggested size of poster(s): 8½ X 11, 14 X 17 (Consider they must be transported.)
3.) Use of lightweight poster board, foam core, or cloth covered poster display board.
4.) Size of lettering: 3/8", 1" or larger.
5.) Diagrams need to be clear and simple.
6.) If you desire a standard format for placement on the board, include a diagram. May include abstract number, title, author(s), sequence or grouping of tables and figures.

Location of session:

1.) Room number or area of convention hall.
2.) Type of board (i.e., fiberboard), type of material to affix (pins, thumbtacks, tape).

Equipment:

1.) Standard equipment is board surface and something to attach poster, or table top display.
2.) Presenter should be told that nothing further is provided if that is the case (i.e., table, projection equipment, pens, paper).

**Suggestions for Presenters**

- Obtain written instructions (well in advance of preparation of presentation) regarding preparation of posters, format, location, and equipment.
- Follow ALL instructions from the conference planners.
- Pointers for presenters include:

Preparation of posters:

1.) Strive for concise, clear posters.
2.) Include all necessary information but nothing unnecessary.
3.) Emphasis is more important than creative art.
4.) Illustrations (charts, tables, diagrams) should be simple and bold.
5.) Sequence your materials (numbers, letters, arrows).
6.) Follow schematic format if provided, otherwise diagram your own.
7.) Poster(s) should be self explanatory so you are free for discussion.
8.) It may be worth it to have someone skilled in visual media to prepare your visuals.

Use of poster:

1.) You may wish to have duplicates (scaled down) of some part of poster board illustrations or supplementary handouts (i.e., abstract, bibliographies).
2.) Avoid damage to board surface by following instructions for methods of attaching posters to the board. Use the correct type of pin or tape. Use Velcro to attach items to cloth display boards.
3.) Set up and take down your poster display at the designated times.
4.) Incorporate evaluation of the poster board session in your planning.

**Other Related Methodologies:** Poster Session, Poster Presentation.

## References


Bauer, E. How to use poster boards at medical meetings. (1979, September). Medical Meetings, 6 (4), 70-71.

Craig, J. F., & Moreland, E. F. (1978, January). Short Subjects. Biomedical Communications, 6 (1), 24-25. (Use of mini-workshops for faculty to encourage them to use media in dentistry.)

Gustafson, M. (1981, March/April). Poster presentation -- More than a poster on a board! The Journal of Continuing Education in Nursing 12 (2), 28-30.

Morra, M. E. (1984, March/April). How to plan and carry out your poster session. Oncology Nursing Forum, 11 (2), 52-57.

Sexton, D. L. (1984, Nov./Dec.). Presentation of research findings: The poster session. Nursing Research, 33 (6), 374-375.

Van Hoozer, H. (1982). Designing and producing scientific and educational posters. Visual Communication Basic Guidelines (pp. 40-50). Iowa City, IA: The University of Iowa.

# PROCESS RECORDING

## Definition

*Process Recording* is the verbatim, serial reproduction of the verbal and nonverbal communications between two individuals for the purpose of assessing the interactions.

## Purposes

- Provide a systematic record of the verbal and nonverbal communication between two individuals, which may be examined, analyzed, and evaluated.
- Provides useful identification of the learning needs of the individual student.
- Provides opportunity for learner to gain awareness of his/her own communication and its effect on others.
- Permits written exchange of ideas between teachers and learners; may be supplemented by other methods, such as audio tape or conference.

---

## Advantages

- Process recording provides a permanent record of growth over time.
- It is a useful teaching tool in all three domains -- cognitive, affective, psychomotor.
- It may be combined with audio tape and videotape for greater accuracy and detail.
- It may be a useful tool for both one-to-one interactions and large groups in a clinical setting.

## Disadvantages

- If transcribed from memory, much of both verbal and nonverbal communication may be missing or unintentionally distorted, leading to inaccurate perception and analysis.
- For some learners, it may be more difficult to note and record nonverbal communication at the same time they are focusing on verbal communication.
- Time consuming.
- Tape recordings (most accurate and complete, except for videotaping or use of two-way mirror observation) require even more time of both student and faculty member.
- Commentary may be delayed and difficult for the student to understand and utilize in revisions.

---

## Points to Remember

- Correlate use of tool with class and individual goals.
- Give complete, explicit instructions (probably best if they are written and given well in advance of when the first record is to be submitted).

- List in instructions the parts of the process recording (written record, feelings, analysis) and its format.
- Plan when, how often, and how records are to be submitted and returned to the student, and explain the use of the teacher's comments and any action expected.
- Indicate whether grading or only evaluation will be involved.
- Consider the use of contract grading if appropriate.
- Consider combination with other means -- audio taping, videotaping, etc.
- Plan for evaluation of the use of the teaching method.
- Prepare and seek permission of client or second individual, when appropriate.
- Combine individual's record with conferences before and after.
- Encourage honesty and openness and support students in their sharing.
- Have a specific purpose; do not overuse the method.

**References**

Baker, J., Pelto, C., & Wittman, E. (1976). An alternative to process recording. Nursing Outlook, 24(2), 115-118. (A faculty member and two students in a psycho social nursing course discuss direct observation as an alternative and tell why they preferred that approach.)

Cosper, B. (1976). Coping with an increased student-faculty ratio. American Journal of Nursing, 76(10), 1642-1644. (A teacher in a baccalaureate program shares four techniques helpful in guiding large groups of students through clinical experience -- one of which is the process recording.)

Nehren, J.G., & Batey, M. (1963). The process recording -- A method of teaching interpersonal relationship skills. Nursing Forum, 2(2), 65-73. (Specific format and use of the teaching tool, for development of interpersonal relationship skills).

Schweer, J. E., & Gebbie, K. (1976). Creative teaching in clinical nursing(3rd ed., pp. 122-124). St. Louis: C.V. Mosby. (Suggests very specific procedure to follow in use of the method; and indicates that it can be used broadly in clinical teaching by a knowledgeable teacher.)

# PROJECTS

## Definition

*Projects* is a significant, practical unit of activity having educational value and aimed at one or more definite goals of understanding, involves investigation and solution of problems, and frequently, the use and manipulation of physical materials, planned and carried to completion by learners and teacher in a natural, "real life" manner.

## Purposes

- Permits student to prepare a product of educational value.
- Provide for experiential learning.
- Provide an alternative form of homework.
- Share with peers and clients the results of investigation and/or manipulation.

---

**Advantages**

- Allows for individual initiative.
- Provides for display of creative and unique interests of learners.
- Allows variety in presentations of group of learners.
- Provides activities for groups of various sizes.
- Assists in learning selected psychomotor skills by discovery method.

**Disadvantages**

- Could become expensive and very time consuming.
- Learners may need criteria, guidelines, and equipment.
- Without a careful plan, would emphasize product rather than process.

---

## Points to Remember

- Select and plan for projects that are consistent with course objectives.
- Provide criteria, guidelines, and materials as appropriate.
- Differentiate evaluation and grading of projects.
- Set limits for expenditure of materials, time and energy.

**Other Related Methodologies:** Homework, Exhibits, Learning Fair.

## References


Hall, B. (1961). Projects -- A teaching method. Nursing Time, 57, 1096-1098.

Podratz, R. O. (1976). Audio-visual project: An alternative learning experience in pediatrics. Journal of Nursing Education, 15(6), 33-36.

Yens, D. (1963). The project method. American Journal of Nursing, 36(2), 174-176.

## PROVERB

### Definition

*Proverb* is a brief, pithy saying, condensing in witty or striking form the wisdom of experience; a familiar and widely known popular saying in epigrammatic form.

### Purpose

- Mechanism for information processing
- Give instruction
- Sum up argument

---

**Advantages**

- Universal form of oral tradition.
- In many cultures, as a person progresses to status of elder in a community, he/she knows more numbers of proverbs and times to use them.
- Easy to remember due to short, concise nature.

**Disadvantages**

- Requires knowledge of culture and language.
- Societal rules govern use (i.e., in some areas, it is disrespectful for youngsters to quote an adult).

---

### Points to Remember

- May be difficult to locate those that pertain to the topic area to be studied.
- User may or may not know how and when to use.

### References


Balutansky, K. (1977). (Editor and translator). Tambour Battant, Goshen, IN: Pinchpenny Press, Goshen College.

Fugelsand, A. (1979, October). Beans in a bowl. Development Communication Report (USAID #28, pp. 8-9), Washington, DC.

Kin, D. (Ed.). (1955). Dictionary of American proverbs. New York: Philosophical Library.

Stevenson, B. (1965). The Macmillan book of proverbs, maxims and famous phrases. New York: Macmillan Co.

# PUPPETS

## Definition

*Puppet* is an inanimate form that is operated by a person, before an audience, to communicate an idea. A specialized form of dramatization.

## Purposes

- Stimulates interest and involvement.
- Teaches facts and concepts by helping to make the abstract concrete.
- Arouses curiosity and involves imagination.
- Entertains by telling stories.
- Encourages expression of thoughts and feelings.
- Helps groups of learners to teach each other and work together, as in presenting a puppet show.
- Evokes emotion.

---

## Advantages

- Puppets can present ideas effectively with extreme simplicity.
- Puppets can do things that real actors cannot.
- Puppets can deal with critical or controversial subject matter.
- They provide elements of fun and surprise.
- Puppets are useful for any age and almost any place.
- They are versatile -- almost anything can be "personalized."
- They are inexpensive -- almost any item can become a puppet, including throwaway items.
- They are mobile and portable -- may be carried in a pocket or hidden in a drawer.
- They are simple to use and to make.
- They may be used by an individual or group.

## Disadvantages

- Teacher may forget it is the movement of the puppet that "makes it great."
- Puppets may be overused.
- They may be expensive.
- More elaborate puppet shows may require much time and effort.

---

## Suggestions for Use in Health Care

Assessment. To win confidence, decrease fear or antagonism toward health personnel, establish trust and rapport, ask and/or answer questions, arouse.

Intervention. Through allaying fears and anxieties, the learner is able to listen and learn, impart information via directions and/or instructions, explain what to expect in an exam or procedure, reeducate on health matters where it is necessary to correct misconceptions. To reassure, set a pleasant tone, encourage, compliment, or give positive reinforcement. Use puppets to introduce new people and procedure. Allow learner to manipulate the puppet to show correct position.

Evaluation. Ask questions, stimulate thinking, and review learning. Praise or restate learning or actions.

## Points to Remember

- The thing the puppet does best is move. Let movements be bold and deliberate.
- Give your audience a chance to see the message.
- Vary movements; repetition gets monotonous.
- Remember: You control the form, identify, movement, and voice.
- Begin to look for ordinary objects at home and in health-care settings that can be used as puppets.
- Experiment with handy object to start with -- a pencil, piece of chalk.
- Familiarize yourself with the major types of puppets and read idea books for easy ways to make or sources for purchase (see Wilt et al.).
- Practice with the puppet prior to the presentation.
- Seek learner evaluation of your use of the method.

## Types of Puppets

- Hand and finger puppets. These are the most immediate types. With finger puppets, some type of head is placed on the puppeteer's finger or fingers. There are no strings or rods, no moving parts that might break or tangle, and no controls to fool with. Hand puppets may be ready-made or can be made from many things -- glove, paper bag, envelope, sock, Styrofoam ball, felt, fruit, vegetable.
- Rod puppets. Any object to which you can attach a stick or rod can become a rod puppet. It may be "personalized" with features and costume may be made from cardboard tube, egg beater, surgical instrument, stuffed paper bag, tongue blade.
- Shadow puppets. An ancient art form; the audience does not see the puppet, only its shadow cast on a screen. Lends itself to much experimentation with shapes, colors, textures, and screens. Bright light shining from back of screen is necessary.

- String puppets, or marionettes. A stick and a ball on a string can become a marionette. Flat forms may have strings added, as well as two- or three-dimensional objects. A stage may be made from a folding table placed on its side, two chairs, a swerving window, or a large box, e.g., one in which a refrigerator was packed.
- Whole-costume puppet. Some of the best known are the Walt Disney characters, with individuals in costume acting as puppets.

**References**


Bard, B. (1965). The art of the puppet. New York: MacMillan. (Books with many colored photographs of puppets; a documentary of puppets throughout the ages. Bill and Cora Baird assisted Indian educators in the use of puppets for instruction in health.)

Cassell, S., & Paul, M. H. (1967). The role of puppet therapy on the emotional responses of children hospitalized for cardiac catheterization. Journal of Pediatrics, 71(2), 233-239. (A research study showing the value of puppets in therapy.)

Gustafson, M. (1980). Puppets in the nursing process. Supervisor Nurse, 11(11), 33-35.

Holmes, A. C. (1964). Health education in developing countries (pp. 102-196). Camden, NJ: Nelson. (Specific suggestions for using puppets in health education.)

Johnson, B. H. (1974). Before hospitalization: A preparation program for the child and his family. Children Today, 3(6), 18-21.

Ka, K. D. (1982). Using puppets to teach ideas. Development Communication Report (#40, pp. 3-4).

Kinder, J. S. (1959). Audio-visual materials and techniques (2nd ed.). New York: American Book Company. (A valuable chart on p. 510 indicates the various types of puppets most appropriate to various age levels from kindergarten through ninth grade.)

Kinder, J. S. (1973). Using instructional media (pp. 170-173). New York: D. Van Nostrand. (Basic material on the use of puppets in education.)

Meehan, T. (1980). Puppets are people, disabled but not different. Biomedical Communication, 9(6) 18-19.

Norberta, Sister. (1976). Caring for children with the help of puppets. American Journal of Maternal Child Nursing, 1(1), 22-26. (Illustrates a pediatric nurse practitioner's use of hand puppets.)

# ROLE-PLAY

## Definition

*Role Playing* is the assuming, either in imagination or overtly, the part of another or others.

## Purposes

- Develop interpersonal skills -- mutual respect, acceptance, and expression of feelings.
- Present content in the affective domain.
- Try alternative approaches and examine the consequences of alternative approaches.
- Experience and describe the thoughts and feelings of participants in a situation by assuming that role.
- Trigger further questions and ideas from learners.
- Introduce and develop concepts through active discovery.

---

**Advantages**

- Inexpensive in terms of equipment and facilities.
- May be used spontaneously.
- Most useful in teaching in affective domain.
- Possibilities are limitless in both teaching and evaluation.
- May tailor materials to needs and interests of your class.
- Practice in reality and risk "making mistakes."
- Allows for risk taking and mistake making.

**Disadvantages**

- May pressure and/or embarrass learners.
- Requires planning and preparation by teacher, as well as skillful use in many situations.
- Tends to be used without caution to basic rules.
- To use role playing you need time -- especially to discuss the playing.
- Role playing is a method, not an end in itself.

---

## Responsibilities of Teacher

- Establish the group -- define the problem or create readings.
- Choose participants -- from volunteers.
- Instruct participants -- and perhaps the observers.
- Stop or cut the situations -- 3-6 minutes is usually adequate.
- Interpret situations -- analysis, discussion, evaluation.

## Format

- Teacher should bring a well-structured, but brief, problem which does not have too direct a relationship to the learners own personal problems.
- Situation should be one which is familiar enough so members understand roles and their potential responses to the problem.
- Role-players should participate voluntarily.
- Role-playing is not to be rehearsed; is not a skit.
- Brief time may be provided for players to prepare -- think about their role, not to rehearse, but to "get into role."
- Assigning names to the players further helps to get them "in role."
- It may be helpful to have written instructions (brief).
- May wish to assign observers to identify with some specific roles and/or players.
- Players are asked to discuss situation before the observers do.
- Direct discussion away from reactions of participants to reactions of people in general.

## Variations

- Reverse roles.
- Two or more presentations of same situation may be used to illustrate different views.

**Other Related Methodologies:** Psychodrama, Skit, Simulation game.

## References Used For Guideline Development


Chesler, M., & Fox, R. (1966). Role-playing methods in the classroom. Chicago: Science Research Associates.

DePablo, S., & Acherhalt, E. (1978). Teaching the use of restraint through role play. Perspectives in Psychiatric Care, 16(5-6), 218-222.

Good, C. V. (1973). Dictionary of Education (3rd ed.). New York: McGraw-Hill Book Co.

Gordon, I., et al. (1969). Role playing as a technique for teaching medical students. Journal of Medical Education, 35, 781-785.

Klein, A. F. (1965). Role-playing in leadership training and group problem solving New York: Association Press. (One of the more complete books on the use of the method.)

McKeachie, W. (1969). Teaching tips: A guidebook for the beginning college teacher (6th ed.). Lexington, MA: D. C. Health & Co. (Briefly outlines and uses the teachers' responsibilities.)

# SELF LEARNING PACKETS

**Definition**

*Self Learning Packets* are free standing learning activities that can be done by the learner without an instructor present.

**Purposes**

- Allow for self paced learning.
- Provide education needed for one individual at the time when they need it.

---

**Advantages**

- Flexible, timely learning.
- Can take on many forms -- video tapes, reading materials, slide-tape activities, etc.
- Self-paced learning.
- Ideal for one person or small groups.
- Cost effective for material taught more than one time.

**Disadvantages**

- May be confusing to learner if objectives and instructions are not well defined.
- Not cost effective for material taught only once.

---

**Points to Remember**

- Self Learning Packet should be well defined. Include the following in each packet:
  - Title
  - Brief description
  - Audience it is intended for
  - Length of activity
  - Instructions for completion
  - Where to return material
- Update and revise materials as needed.
- Self learning activities can be very cost effective. Most of the cost is up front, very little ongoing costs to maintain. Self learning is not cost effective for something taught only once.

**References**


Cooper, S. (1986). Teaching tips: Self-directed learning. Journal of Continuing Education in Nursing, 17 (3), May/June, 104-105.

Wright, D. (1996). How to create and promote self learning packets (videotape) Minneapolis, MN: Creative HealthCare Management.

Yarnall, Nikolajski P. (1992). Investigating the effectiveness of self-learning packages in staff development. Journal of Nursing Staff Development July/August, 1992. 179-183.

# SEMINAR

## Definition

*Seminar* is a group of learners which meets under the general direction of one or more leaders for a discussion of problems or mutual interests.

## Purposes

- Provides opportunity for careful study under the guidance of a well-qualified authority.
- Arrives at a conclusion founded on thorough investigation and research.
- Presents information systematically.
- Discusses information necessary for the solution of a problem.
- Identifies and explores problems.

---

**Advantages**

- Learners share information and challenge each other's ideas.
- Active participation is stimulated in the discussion of information.
- Careful, systematic inquiry and debate can occur.
- Activity is guided by a recognized authority.

**Disadvantages**

- It is often difficult to obtain a person with necessary qualifications to direct the seminar.
- Members may not spend the time required for preparing adequately.
- Appropriate resources may not be available.
- Members may be reluctant to participate verbally in the presence of an expert.
- It is often difficult to develop an idea fully within a limited time period.
- Members must have ability to comprehend topic and be somewhat similar in background.

---

## Format

- The leader(s) is chosen for his or her extensive knowledge in the topic and ability to assist others to learn.
- Seminar members usually are persons with similar knowledge and background. They should be interested in the topic and willing to undertake systematic, thoughtful study and discussion.

## Responsibilities

Leader:

a. Prior to seminar

(1) Plans with needs and interests of members in mind.

(2) Make arrangements for necessary materials and facilities.
(3) Suggests advance preparation to members.
(4) Assigns readings and suggests provocative discussion questions.
(5) Seeks to clarify purpose and goals of the seminar.
(6) Considers techniques, devices, and educational aids to be used for presenting information and promoting discussion.
(7) Prepares introductory speech.

b. During seminar
   (1) Presents introductory speech.
   (2) Tries to communicate enthusiasm and interest as well as ideas.
   (3) Leads or directs someone else to lead the question period.
   (4) Asks for prepared reports or research.
   (5) Avoids acting exclusively as a teacher -- the ideal is a teaching-learning relationship in which all are learning together.
   (6) Offers resource information on request or at appropriate times.
   (7) Encourages different points of view.
   (8) Helps members to select individual topics for future study.
   (9) Assists each member in preparing his or her report/information.
   (10) Comments on each report and leads a discussion following each report.
   (11) Encourages continued study after the close of the seminar.
   (12) Oversees the arrangement and reproduction of findings in a report (if appropriate).

<u>Seminar members</u>

a. Prior to seminar
   (1) Study and think in preparation, based on goals of the seminar.
   (2) Prepare clear, logical reports.
   (3) Prepare to make contributions to the seminar.

b. During seminar
   (1) Accept responsibility for individual participation in the seminar.
   (2) Select specific topics for individual study.
   (3) Present reports clearly and logically.
   (4) Help the leader and other learners trough active listening and participation.

## Suggestions for Use

- Group may number from 5 to 50, usually about 30.
- Members will need to know how time in the total session is divided among members' reports, question periods, and other activities.
- Environmental comfort will add much to group participation and learning.

## References

Baron, A. (1977). How to start a seminar. <u>Training and Development Journal, 31</u>(12), 22-27. (Suggestions for ice breakers to start a seminar.)

Bergevin, P., Morris, D., & Smith, R. M. (1963). Adult education procedures (pp. 147-157). New York: Seabury Press.

Morgan, B., Holmes, G. E., & Bundy, C. E. (1976). Methods in adult education (3rd ed., pp. 72). Danville, IL: Interstate Printers and Publishers.

Rubin, F., Allan, J. D., & Leak, A. G. (1971). The seminar process -- an aid to learning. Nursing Outlook, 19(1), 37-39.

## Definition

*Simulation* is the use of objects, persons, or environments to represent original reality in highly modified fashion. Some examples of simulations include -- mock emergency events and computer simulations, as well as activities that use simulator devices such as a cardiopulmonary simulator in a CPR mannequin.

## Purposes

- Provides practice in representative real-life situations without danger.
- Reduces training time.
- Provides on-the-job training in skills and procedures not easily acquired through reading or lectures.
- Fosters skill, confidence, and enthusiasm.
- Permits analysis of an event while it is happening.
- Makes a learning experience available to a large number of learners.

---

## Advantages

- Simulation simplifies the instructional process.
- It is less dangerous, costly, and impractical.
- Patients are spared discomfort and/or harm.
- It is possible to plan a gradual increase in the severity and complexity of problems to be solved.
- Single steps may be repeated if necessary.
- Students participate actively while proceeding at individual rates.
- Research supports the value of the method.
- It is widely used in medicine, business, and industry.

## Disadvantages

- Transfer of learning from simulation to a real-life situation is not well documented.
- Simulation may result in distorting, obscuring, or confusing real-life circumstances.
- Learner may have difficulty integrating instruction into real-life situation, since simulations use only selected aspects of reality.
- Simulator devices may be expensive to purchase.
- Teacher and assistants must be knowledgeable and skilled in operating the simulator devices and explaining how it works.
- Simulator devices may require large areas for use and/or storage.
- Simulations are time-consuming to construct and maintain.

---

**Characteristics**

- Simulation attempts to represent a real situation in which operations are carried out.
- Simulation provides users with certain controls over that situation.
- Simulation is deliberately designed to omit certain parts of real operational situations that are not important for the particular training or are too dangerous, impractical, or expensive to represent.

**Other Related Methodologies:** Gaming, Computer Simulations, Demonstration.

**References**


Barrows, H. (1972). Simulated patients. Springfield, IL: Charles C. Thomas. (One of the first to use simulated patients in medical education describes their selection, preparation, and use.)

Cooper, S. (1979). Methods of teaching -- Revisited. Games and simulation. Journal of Continuing Education in Nursing, 10 (5), 14+.

Dale, E. (1969). Audiovisual methods in teaching (3rd ed., pp. 235-240). New York: Dryden Press, Holt, Rinehart & Winston. (Basic information on simulations in teaching.)

Gilbert, G. G. (1975, June). A working model for simulation techniques. Health Education, 6 (3), 10-13. (Simulated situations were used to teach emergency care.)

Godkins, R. R., Duffy, D., & Stanhope, W. D. (1974). Utilization of simulated patient to teach routine pelvic examination to new health practitioners. P.A. Journal, 4 (2), 26-31. (A report of the use of simulated patients in medical education to teach routine pelvic examinations.)

Gordon, M. S. (1975). Learning from a cardiology patient simulator. RN, 38 (8), ICU-1-ICU-6. (A physician describes the computer-programmed animated manikins for teaching health/medical students.)

Lincoln, R. E., Layton, J., & Holdman, H. (1978). Using simulated patients to teach assessment. Nursing Outlook, 26 (5), 316-320.

Pearson, B. D. (1975). Simulation techniques for nursing education. International Nursing Review, 22 (5), 144-146. (Purposes, uses and value of simulation techniques in nursing education.)

Story, D. (1972). A mock disaster on a rural road. American Journal of Nursing, 72 (12), 2222-2224. (A mockup, one form of simulation, used by students in two programs in Iowa.)

Hoban, D. (1978). Successful simulations for health education. Audiovisual Instruction, 23 (9), 20-22.

Kolb, S., & Shugart, E. (1984). Evaluation: Is simulation the answer? Journal of Nursing Education, 23 (2), 84-86.

Laszlo, S., & McKenzie, J. (1979). The use of a simulation game in training hospital staff about patient rights. Journal of Continuing Nursing Education, 10 (5), 30-36.

Lehrer, S. (1980). The professional patient session as a technique for teaching the GYN exam to nurse practitioner students. Journal of Nursing Education, 19 (5), 39-47.

McDowell, J., et al. (1984). Evaluating clinical performance using simulated patients. Journal of Nursing Education, 1, 37-39.

McGuire, C. H. (1978). Evaluation of clinical performance: Written and oral simulations. In A. G. Rezlek & B. J. Stevens (Eds.), The nurse evaluator in education and service (pp. 101-124.

Newman, M. A., & O'Brien, R. A. (1978). Experiencing the research process via computer simulation. Image, 10 (1), 5-9. (The computer as a dynamic teaching tool.)

Page, G. G. (1978). Written simulation in nursing. Journal of Nursing Education, 17 (4), 28-32. (Written simulations as an adjunct to other methods in clinical teaching.)

# SKETCHING

## Definition

*Sketching* is to draw, describe, or outline chief features of a person, object, or place.

## Purposes

- Communicates visual knowledge.
- Suggests a point.
- Provides an image -- either visually or mentally.
- Adds interest and clarity to posters, chalkboards, transparencies, stories, tape recordings.

---

**Advantages**

- No artistic ability is required.
- Teacher and students may draw their own ideas.
- Since the rough drawing presents only the chief features, learners fill in gaps with their own imagination.
- There are books available that teach simple, step-by-step figure drawings.

**Disadvantages**

- Sketching is generally believed to require artistic talent.
- Teachers and students are often afraid to try.

---

## Points to Remember

- Simplicity is the most important.
- Drawing should be large, bold, simple, and "free" -- informal, and spontaneous.
- Start with stick figures and simple cartoons.
- As skills develop, explore three-dimensional forms and strive for technical accuracy.
- Use books that teach how to sketch (Davidow, Pigrem, and Thompson).
- Practice on a chalkboard, a transparency, and other media.

## References

Brown, J., et al. (1969). A-V instruction materials and methods (3rd ed.). New York: McGraw-Hill. (How to combine sketching with the chalkboard and storytelling.)

Dale, E. (1969). Audiovisual methods in teaching (3rd ed., pp. 511-512). New York: Dryden Press, Holt, Rinehart & Winston.

Davidow, A. (1977). Let's draw animals. New York: Gosset & Dunlap. (An inexpensive paperback that gives simple, step-by-step instructions for drawing animals.)

Hord, E. (1981). Drawing on your resources. Biomedical Communications, 9(4), 18-20.

Pigrem, S. (1977). Help I can't draw. Minneapolis: Augsburg Publishing House. (A series of three paperbacks that tell how to make visuals to use in religious education.)

Thompson, K. (1978). Sketching and telling stories to children. Grand Rapids, MI: Zondervan Publishing House. (Instructions on how to sketch illustrations for religious education.)

# SLIDE

## Definition

*Slide* is a relatively small piece of film or other transparent material on which a single pictorial or graphic image has been placed for still projection on to a wall or screen.

## Purposes

- Projects still pictures at a rate that can be varied to keep pace with comments of the teacher and questions from learners.
- Communicates to viewers a common experience upon which to build discussion.
- Helps teach process and procedures.
- Motivates students not secure in verbal work.

---

## Advantages

- Slides are convenient to use, easy to obtain in high quality, relatively inexpensive, and easy to make.
- A great variety of images can be depicted.
- Projector is cheaper than movie projector or video projector.
- Slides are useful for almost any age group.

They may be used for individual study or large groups.

## Disadvantages

- Slides need to be projected large enough to be seen by all.
- The larger and/or more numerous the slides, the more storage area is required.
- Each presentation requires filing, storage, and organizing slides.

---

## Suggestions for Preparing

- A slide can be made of anything that is drawn, painted, written, typewritten, printed, or photographed.
- Keep it simple -- no more than five or six lines per slide.

## Suggestions for Purchasing

- There are many commercial sources. Select wisely.
- There are title slides available for purchase (Title Slides, Inservice Magazine, Dept. S., Suite 1306, 60 E. 42nd St., New York, NY, 10017).

## Points to Remember

- Use a tabletop slide viewer to select slides.
- Group slides according to sequence of ideas.

- Make your final choices only after trial projection on a screen.
- Write or rewrite script in direct relationship to pictures.
- Determine what title, captions, and other artwork will be needed.
- Use a large number of slides and move them quickly.
- Be well prepared with audio accompaniment, questions, comments, and explanations.
- Review and rehearse.
- Check electrical equipment and screen placement.
- Make sure room can be darkened sufficiently.

**Other Related Methodologies:** Filmstrip, Slide-tape.

**References**


Bauer, E. J. (1977). The KISS principle for speaker slide preparation: Keep it simple, stupid! Medical Meetings, 4(3), 32. (A practical article about slide presentations.)

Eastman Kodak Company. Effective lecture slides (Kodak Pamphlet 8-22). Rochester, NY: Author. (May be useful for those wanting to make their own slides.)

Homemade slides-tapes are a bargain, but.... (1973, Jan./Feb.). Inservice Education and Training, 3(1), 49-53.

Kinder, J. S. Using instructional media (pp. 69-75). New York: D. Van Nostrand.

Schmalenberg, C. (1979). Making and using slides. Nurse Educator, 4(4), 12-15.

Stewart, P. (1981). Utilizing slides in the learning experience. Nurse Educator, 6(4), 9-11.

VanHoozer, H. (1982). Visual communication basic guidelines. Iowa City, IA: University of Iowa, College of Nursing.

# SLIDE-TAPE

## Definition

*Slide-tape* is audio-visual communication which combines the use of slides and sound (usually audiocassette) for a specific program.

## Purposes

- Combined slides, which present a theme or procedure, with verbal (or musical) accompaniment.
- Inform, instruct, involve.
- Provide step by step education to one or more learners.

---

## Advantages

- Can be specifically prepared by an individual or group, when ready-made materials do not meet specific needs.
- Inexpensive.
- Utilize creative ideas.
- Able to use basic equipment already available.
- Versatile -- for various ages and interest of both patients and staff.
- Can be used for a group or as an audio-tutorial method for one individual.

## Disadvantages

- Requires time.
- Requires organization and planning.
- May become expensive.
- Needs periodic revision and updating.

---

## Equipment Needed

- Simple, reliable slide projector.
- Cassette tape player.
- Camera -- for taking slides.
- Screen (or use slide projector with built in viewer screen).

## Suggestions for Making Homemade Slide-Tape

- Begin with three basic elements of a) objectives, b) description of audience, and c) content outline.
- Write the basic content outline.
- Use story board (or individual index cards) (one story board per slide).
- Edit content by dividing into separate concepts.
- Artwork or photography is probably the largest task. (May use simple instant camera.)

- Develop "running" or "shooting" script.
  a. Audio portion of individual slides should be no longer than 2-3 minutes.
  b. All elements should be presented clearly simple, logically.
  c. Complexity of information should be limited.
  d. Allow 3 seconds of silence between slides if material is of average complexity. Allow more time if more complex.
  e. All slides should be relevant, attractive and easily understood.
  f. Keep all slides in horizontal format.
  g. Ask knowledgeable individual (but not one familiar with the script) to review at this point.
- Obtain necessary permission for use of visual or verbal content.
- Recording:
  a. Use conversational style.
  b. Determine if you wish to have (or not to have) a specific voice.
- Evaluate completed program. Provide for similar evaluation by use of evaluation forms. Use as base for revision and update.

**Points to remember**

- You may have more complex equipment, such as synchronizing tape recorder with inaudible "beep", more than one slide projector, etc.
- Clearly label all slides, tapes, and boxes.
- Keep all written materials used, for later reference.
- Copyright privileges may be important.

**Other Related Methodologies:** Cassette Tape, Slides.

**References**

Burge, S. (1977). Producing an effective slide/tape program. Training and Development Journal, 31(12), 12-13. (A brief article with some specific ideas.)

Homemade slide-tapes are a bargain, but.... (1973, Jan./Feb.). Inservice Education and Training, 3(1), 49-53. (Diploma program nursing instructors describe their uses of slide-tape.)

Your slide show and how to produce it. Rochester, NY: Singer Education Division. (A very useful pamphlet, giving step-by-step instructions.)

# SNAPSHOT

## Definition

*Snapshot* is a candid photograph depicting a moment in time.

## Purposes

- Preserves an instant in time.
- Conveys a great deal of warmth and definition.
- Teaches the steps in a process or procedure.
- Assists in identifying individuals or information.
- Conveys an idea in a picture.

---

## Advantages

- A photograph is a permanent record.
- It may be used in the affective, cognitive, and psychomotor domains.
- It is versatile -- can be used by both learner and teacher.
- It can increase interest in a subject.
- It has a rich supplemental value in teaching.
- It goes beyond physical and temporal limitations.
- It may be combined with other media (audio or other visual methods). Most people have simple, inexpensive cameras at their disposal and some knowledge of how to use them.

## Disadvantages

- Photographs are generally limited to small group use or to some form of enlargement or projection for large groups.
- Poor technical production may detract from their educational value.
- Time is needed to take and develop photographs.
- They may become costly.

---

## Points to Remember

- Relate photographs to learning objective.
- Budget and function will determine the kind of camera, finishing process, and end product.
- There are numerous ways of using photographs in teaching.
- Identification of learners or group members may be facilitated by use of photographs posted or submitted with written assignments.
- Photographs may be used creatively in combination with teaching. (Be sure to follow protocol for permission to take and use, however.)

- Follow criteria for selecting photographs for educational purposes.
  a. Must be educationally useful and the information accurate.
  b. Must show an interpretable message clearly.
  c. Must demonstrate good technical aspects, such as focus, pleasing composition, proper exposure and development (if in color, colors must be true). Message of the photo is the main focus.
- There are books of photographs that may be worth purchasing, such as Gramps or The Family of Man.
- The teacher may find it useful to protect and preserve some photographs by covering and/or framing them.
- Orderly filing and storage will assist in reuse.

**Ideas for Taking Photographs**

- Follow instructions for using the camera.
- Plan the subject matter. Arrange for balance, not necessarily symmetry.
- Keep the picture simple, to aid in understanding and remembering.
- Take close-ups -- they attract attention.
- Keep the subject busy; he or she will generally look more natural that way.
- Watch the background and keep it plain. Avoid extremely light or dark backgrounds.
- Be sure the camera is in focus and adjusted for the proper amount of light.
- Experiment with equipment and supplies.
- If taking photographs involves learners, it may be wise to have printed instructions.
- Instant development cameras may allow for flexibility in learning activity -- there is no time lag between taking photo and development of photo.

**Other Related Methodologies:** Instant Development (Polaroid, Kodak), Photo Story.

**References**

Kinder, J. (1973). Using instructional media (pp. 53-54). New York: D. Van Nostrand. (Although brief, a very useful section on photographs.)

Koch, H. (1975). The static visual media. Nursing Outlook, 23(6), 355. (Lists criteria for selecting photographs.)

Davis, M. (1977). Getting to the root of the problem, Hair grooming techniques for black patients. Nursing '77, 7(4), 60-65.

Gordon, J. (1977). Circoelectric beds, circumventing the trauma of positioning. Nursing '77, 7(2), 42-47.

Murray, J., & Smallwood, J. (1977). CVP monitoring, sidestepping potential perils. Nursing '77, 7(1), 42-47.

# SPECIMENS

**Definition**

*Specimens* are real things treated and thus preserved.

**Purpose**

- To permit seeing and studying real objects that would otherwise be difficult to observe.

---

| | |
|---|---|
| **Advantages** | • Allows learners to classify, draw conclusions, and generalize.<br>• Allows learner to view object thoroughly and more than once. |
| **Disadvantages** | • Storage containers (jars and bottles) may be breakable.<br>• Containers require storage and careful labeling.<br>• May be expensive. |

---

**Other Related Methodologies:** Object Lesson

**References**


Brown, J. W., Lewis, R. B., & Harcleroad, F. (1964). A-V Instruction materials and methods (2nd ed.). New York: McGraw-Hill.

Saunders, D. J. (1979). Visual communication handbook. London: United Society for Christian Literature.

# STORY BOARD

## Definition

*Story Board* is a series of sketches or pictures which visualize a topic. Story boards can be used as an educational/informative display or to organize a script for an audio/visual production.

## Purposes

- Assist in visualization ideas.
- Provides system and assists in overall organization by:
  a. giving designer an integrated overview.
  b. allows for easy sequencing and rearrangement.
  c. allows for easy deletion or replacement.
  d. allows for easy revision or refinement.

---

**Advantages**

- Great way to tell a story or describe a sequence of events.
- Requires little equipment.
- Various types of pictures may be used -- flap pictures, sketches, Polaroid.
- May be used in preparing several visuals -- slides, slide-tape, filmstrip, flap pictures, kamishibai.
- May be developed by an individual or group.

**Disadvantages**

- Is time consuming.
- Learners may not be familiar with story board concepts for development.

---

## Points to Remember

- Technique requires note cards and large wall or table. (There are commercially prepared boards for those who desire).
- May contain visual, production notes, or suggested narration.
- Consider leaving room for narration.
- Leave space for titles, questions, and special directions if appropriate.
- Examine your work.
- Obtain reactions and suggestions from those interested and qualified.

## References

Clark, C. (1978). Classroom skills for nurse educator (pp. 280-290). New York: Springer Publishing Co.

Kemp, J. (1963). Planning and producing audio visual materials(3rd ed., pp. 52-54). New York: Thomas Y. Crowell.

Ledford, B., & Gordon, T. (1976, September). Script card to story board. Audiovisual Instruction, 21(7), 44-45.

**Definition**

*Storytelling* is an oral narration of fact or fiction.

**Purposes**

- Expresses life's meaning, purpose, and heritage via oral tradition.
- Enlivens factual information.
- Demonstrates teacher or learner creativity.
- Puts audience, class, or individual student at ease.

---

**Advantages**

- Storytelling needs no added materials or equipment.
- It involves learners' imaginations.
- It is universally enjoyed by all ages.
- It is a practical cross-cultural method.
- It may be used with people who are unable to read.
- Stories may be combined with visual supplements (chalkboard, flannel board) and audio (cassette).

**Disadvantages**

- Storytelling is an art, and must be studied and practiced by the teacher.
- It requires preparation.
- It is boring to listeners if poorly done.

---

**Points to Remember**

- Listen to expert storytellers.
- Prepare by reading the story in your own words before a mirror and/or record it on tape.
- Practice telling the story in your own words before a mirror and/or record it on tape.
- Pitch story to level of listeners' understanding; be natural, use short sentences and words that are understandable.
- Compare verbal enthusiasm with facial expressions and gestures.
- Correct voice use includes a pleasing pitch, lack of nasality, and frequent changes in inflection.
- Use conversational tones and dialogue.
- Pause before surprise turns; use slow tempo for sad or suspenseful passages, and quicken pace for happy or violent scenes.
- Use good diction at all times.
- Keep it brief for children -- usually 1 minute per year of the child's life (a 4-year-old can listen attentively for 4 minutes).
- With children or those in wheelchairs, sit at eye level.

- End story when you begin to "lose" audience.
- You may wish to permit and/or encourage questions.
- Evaluate audience understanding by asking questions, or have one or several listeners retell all or part of story.
- You may wish to illustrate with sketches, faces, stick figures.
- You may use a chalkboard, flannel board, or flip chart to illustrate.

**Related Form:** Story Reading.

**References**


Barrett, E. (1960). Storytelling, it's easy. Grand Rapids, MI: Zondervan Publishing. (An expert in storytelling tells how she does it.)

Brown, J., et al. (1969). Audio-visual instructional media and methods (3rd ed., pp. 425, 432). New York: McGraw-Hill.

Fox, F. (1975). A need for storytellers. Science Teacher, 42 (4), 12-14. (A science teacher tells why he thinks young people need storytellers to teacher them.)

Hilton, D. (1987). Storytelling for health teaching. Contact, 110, 1-11.

Sawyer, R. (1962). The way of the storyteller. New York: Viking Press. (A well-known expert tells her own development and gives practical suggestions.)

Seaburg, D. I. (1968). Can the ancient art of storytelling be revived? Speech Teacher, 17 (3), 246-249.

Spencer, R. J. (1968). Mastering the art of story telling. Grade Teacher, 85 (5), 80-82.

Werner, D., & Bower, W. (1982). Helping health workers learn. Palo Alto, CA: Hesperian Foundation.

# STRUCTURED CONTROVERSY

## Definition

*Structured Controversy* is an instructional technique based on cooperative group learning, found to be effective in stimulating involvement in societal issues.

## Purposes

- Stimulate learning involvement in issues concerning technology and society.
- Provide the means for managing controversy constructively.
- Stimulates the use of critical thinking skills.

---

**Advantages**

- Prepare learners for higher levels of thinking rather than just technical competence.
- Can be used in a variety of professions (engineering, science and social studies).
- Promote higher achievement and retention, greater searches for information, accurate understanding of perspectives, creative insights, and a positive attitude toward controversy and fellow learners (these have been demonstrated in research studies).
- Increase students' perspective-taking abilities.
- Useful for a wide variety of grade levels, especially adult learners.

**Disadvantages**

- Requires basic knowledge of the method.
- Requires time for the teacher to prepare the issue, obtain documentation on two opposing positions, and orient learners to the process.

---

## Basic Organizational Format for the Teacher -- 3 steps

1. Choose discussion topic. Depends on interests of instructor and purpose of class/course. Criteria for selection:
    a. two well documented opposing positions are available.
    b. students are able to manage content.
2. Prepare instructional materials. Need the following for EACH position
    a. clear description of group task.
    b. description of phases of controversy procedure and collaborative skills to be used during each phase.
    c. definition of position to be advocated with summary of key arguments supporting positions.
    d. resource materials (including bibliography) to provide evidence and elaboration of arguments supporting position to be advocated.

3. <u>Structure the controversy</u>: For success you need skillful group members and heterogeneity of group membership. (Teacher should requires each group to reach consensus and may ask them to submit report on which all members are evaluated). (Provide "Discussion Rules for Participating in an Academic Controversy" from Johnson, D. and Johnson, R., 1988, page 63).

   <u>Discussion Rules</u>:

   - I am critical of ideas, not people.
   - I focus on making the best decision possible, not on "winning."
   - I encourage everyone to participate and master all the relevant information.
   - I listen to everyone's ideas, even if I do not agree.
   - I restate (paraphrase) what someone has said if it is not clear.
   - I first bring out all the ideas and facts supporting both sides and then try to put them together in a way that makes sense.
   - I try to understand both sides of the issue.
   - I change my mind when the evidence clearly indicates that I should do so.

4. <u>Conduct the controversy:</u> Teacher gives learners specific instructions for 5 phases:

   <u>Phase 1</u>: Learn positions: Plan with a partner how to advocate position effectively, read materials supporting your position and plan persuasive presentation.

   <u>Phase 2</u>: Present positions: Present together forcefully and persuasively. Listen and learn opposing position. Take notes and clarify as necessary.

   <u>Phase 3:</u> Discuss the issue: Argue for the position, presenting facts to support your point of view. Listen to opposition and present counter-arguments.

   <u>Phase 4</u>: Reverse perspectives: As a pair, present opposition position as if you were they. Add new facts.

   <u>Phase 5</u>: Reach a decision: Summarize and synthesize best arguments for BOTH points of view. Reach consensus on position supported by facts. Write report with evidence and rationale for synthesis your group has agreed on. Plan time after controversy to process group function and how performance can be enhanced. Highlight specific conflict management skills students need to master.

**<u>Prerequisites to Promoting Constructive Controversy (Five Strategies)</u>:**

<u>Strategy 1:</u> Structure learning activities cooperatively.

a. Controversy must be defined as interesting problems to be solved rather than win-lose situation.
b. Controversy must be valued as opportunity and challenge.
c. Similarities, as well as differences, between positions must be recognized.
d. Information must be accurately communicated.
e. Feelings (as well as information) need to be communicated and responded to.
f. Students must value and respect each other.
g. Students must feel safe enough to challenge each other's ideas and reasoning.

<u>Strategy 2:</u> Ensure that the groups are heterogeneous -- with differences in personality, social class, sex, background, reasoning strategies, ability levels, etc.

Strategy 3: Distribute information relevant to both sides.
Strategy 4: Teach conflict management skills. (May wish to refer to books on that topic.)
Strategy 5: Teach the procedure of rational argument.

**Potential Schedule for Class Period:**

Introduction: 5 minutes
Assign Perspective: 25 minutes (may also further subdivide the time)
Reverse Perspective: 20 minutes
Open Discussion and Decision Making: 15 minutes
Report Preparation: 15 minutes
Evaluation: Additional directions for the group report may be given out, including criteria for evaluation of the group report (i.e., number of points per category).

**Modifications of the Technique:**

The teacher may give a "question" followed by a brief case scenario, objectives, and a task. "Factors to be considered" may be given, as well as a time schedule and written instructions to students (such as the "Discussion Rules" given earlier). Teacher(s) may monitor the use of the process. It may be necessary to use more than one class session and to suggest points that could be used when arguing.

**References**

deTornyay, R. (1990). Editorial: Helping students deal with controversy. Journal of Nursing Education, 29(4), 149.

Johnson, D. W., & Johnson, R. (1988). Critical thinking through structured controversy. Educational Leadership, 45(8), 58-64.

Johnson, D. W., & Johnson, R. (1985). Classroom conflict: Controversy Vs debate in learning groups. American Educational Research Journal, 22, 37-256.

Johnson, D. W., & Johnson, R. (1979). Conflict in the classroom: Controversy and learning. Review of Educational Research, 49, 51-61.

Pederson, C., Duckett, L., & Maruyama, G. (1990). Using structured controversy to promote ethical decision making. Journal of Nursing Education, 29(4), 150-157.

Pederson, C. (1990). A Comparison of Structured Controversy with Lecture in Nursing Education. Doctoral Dissertation, University of Minnesota.

Pederson, C. (1992). Effects of structured controversy on students' perceptions of their skills in discussing controversial issues. Journal of Nursing Education, 31(3), 101-106.

Pederson, C. (1993). Structured controversy versus lecture on nursing students' beliefs about and attitudes toward providing care for persons with AIDS. Journal of Continuing Education in Nursing, 24, 74-81.

Smith, K. (1984). Structured controversies, Engineering Education, 2, 306-309.

# STUDYCADE

## Definition

*Studycade* is a trip or tour intended as a distinct learning experience, and planned and organized for the participants as they travel and study.

## Purposes

- Combines tour with specific goals of participants.
- Permits learners to contribute to planning.
- Makes accessible study topics not available at home.

---

**Advantages**

- Time of the studycade is convenient to the learners' schedules.
- The tour provides learning in actual situations.
- Some details of the tour are taken care of by others.
- Learning occurs during trip/tour as well as after.

**Disadvantages**

- Tour may be costly.
- Group interests may come before those of individual learners.
- A tour requires much planning and organizing.
- It requires pre-travel study for maximum learning.
- It may require decision to attend far in advance of actual departure date.

---

## Points to Remember

- Participants need to enroll in advance and probably make down payment.
- Participants need to contribute to plans and meet to discuss them.
- An advance reading list, as well as discussion groups along the way, needs to be arranged.
- Someone needs to take care of details of chartered bus, housing, and various regulations depending on tour or trip planned.

**Other Related Methodologies:** Study Tour, Travel Abroad, Field Trip

## References

Gorney-Fadiman, M. (1981). New perspective in continuing education: Travel education. Journal of Continuing Education in Nursing 12(4), 30-33.

Knowles, M. (1970). The modern practice of adult education (p. 155). New York: Associated Press.

# STUDY GUIDE QUESTIONS

## Definition

*Study Guide Questions* are the listing of questions to be used in a study guide discussion.

## Purposes

- Enrich learning by provoking thought and interest.
- Give structure to assigned readings.
- Promote application of knowledge.
- Guide observations (i.e., activities, films, videos).
- Aid organization and learning of materials.

---

**Advantages**

- Enliven discussion.
- Indicates aspects considered important by the teacher.
- Can serve as effective guides to discussion.
- Focus discussion on major points.
- Provides a "take-home," self-paced approach to preparation.

**Disadvantages**

- Structures thinking to teacher's rather than learner's ideas.
- May lead to less creativity in group response.
- Requires careful preparation and/or selection by the teacher/leader.

---

## Responsibilities

Teacher:

1. Need to be concerned with the preparation of questions which are clear, accurate, and appropriate in level, type, and sequence.
2. May be copied and distributed in advance or at beginning of class (or written on chalkboard or overhead).
3. If prepared study questions are a feature of a textbook, teacher will need to determine if and how to use them.

Student:

1. Know how the questions will be used (prior to and during discussion).
2. Group members may wish and/or be asked to determine priority for discussion.

**Other Related Methodologies:** Discussion, Seminar.

**References**

Klevens, C. (1972). Materials and methods and adult education (pp. 225-227). New York: Klevens Publ.

Kotaska, J., & Dickinson, G. (1975). Effects of a study guide on independent adult learning. Adult Education, 25, 161-168.

McKeachie, W. (1978). Teaching tips (7th ed.). Lexington, MA: Health Co.

Morgan, B., Holmes, G., & Bundy, C. (1976). Methods in adult education (3rd ed.). Danville, IL: The Interstate.

## SYLLABUS

**Definition**

*Syllabus* is a condensed outline or statement of main points of a course of study (or of books or other documents).

**Purposes**

- Inform all students where the course is "going."
- Serves as a legal, written contract between instructor and students.
- Guides the shaping of students' learning in accordance with the teacher's expectations.

---

**Advantages**

- Directs students and teachers toward a common goal.
- Encourages and facilitates students' success.

**Disadvantages**

- Requires careful planning and time expenditure.
- When instructor wishes to change, it should be clearly communicated in writing.

---

**Examples of Components of a Model Syllabus:**

Personal information
Course name, code number, number of credits, days-times-location of course. Instructor's name, office location, hours, and phone number (and any restrictions).

Course description
Brief, corresponding to official catalog description. Prerequisites.

Course objectives
What is expected to be achieved, may be general or specific, short term or terminal objectives.

Course calendar
Relevant dates, topic, lectures, readings, projects, and exams. (Changes made during the course should be supplied as new information to the students in writing.)

Course requirements
What is to be done and what are to be evaluated -- homework, attendance, class participation, quizzes, exams.

Texts and other materials
Required and or recommended -- for purchase, "on reserve" in the library, or provided as handouts.

Course grading
What percentage for each activity (exams, reports, homework, journal, lab work, etc.)

Caveat

End with a caveat that protects the instructor and the department if changes need to be made during course. (Example, "subject to change in event of extenuating circumstances.")

**Other Related Methodologies:** Annotated Bibliography, Handouts.

**References**


Altman, H. (1989). Syllabus "Shares what the teacher wants." The Teaching Profession, 3(5), 1-2.

de Tornyay, R., & Thompson, M. (1987). Strategies for teaching nursing (3rd ed., pp. 79-86). New York: John Wiley & Sons.

Paduano, M. (1975). The greening of the classroom. Journal of Nursing Education, 14(2), 20-24.

# SYMPOSIUM

**Definition**

*Symposium* is a series of related speeches by 2-5 persons qualified to speak with authority on different phases of the same or closely related topics.

**Purposes**

- Present information in an organized way.
- Reveal a wide range of authoritative opinion about a controversial topic or issue.
- Permit analysis of several related aspects of a controversial topic.
- Clarify closely related problems.
- Assist people to understand the relationships of various parts of a topic to the whole topic.
- Stimulated fresh thinking by people who tend to have similar interests and background.

---

**Advantages**

- Several short speeches prevent boredom and stimulate listening.
- Guard against oversimplification and distortion since various aspects are required to be covered.
- Audience benefits from wide range of knowledge, experience and opinions.
- Considerable amount of information can be shared.
- Encourages each speaker to carefully prepare to speak for a limited time and to stay on the topic.

**Disadvantages**

- Audience may drift into passive moods.
- Speakers may fail to check with each other and result in repetition of information and deviations from the assigned topic.
- Does not permit active audience participation.
- If chairperson is weak, general confusion may result.

---

**Points to Remember**

- Chairperson presides, sets the stage, calls on experts (and keeps each speaker within the time limits), and sees that the speeches are interrelated.
- Speakers need to be well informed and capable of making relatively brief (3-20 minutes), logical presentations that take into account the needs and interests of the audience. The speakers do not converse with each other.
- Preplanning involves careful choice of chairperson and presenters, where topics and details are spelled out clearly and well in advance. (Further details for the method may be found in the guidelines for "guest speaker" and "panel".)

## Alternative Form

The ancient form of the symposium involved 5-20 persons who met in a home or private dining room to enjoy food, entertainment and discuss informally a topic of mutual interest. The moderator was a symposiarch.

## References


Bergevin, P., Morris, D., & Smith, R. (1963). Adult education procedures. New York: Seabury Press.

Morgan, B., Holmes, G., & Bundy, C. (1976). Methods in adult education (3rd ed.). Danville, IL: The Interstate Publishers.

# TALK SHOW

## Definition

*Talk show* is a form of interviewing and discussion demonstrated on several TV talk program. (Phil Donahue Show, Oprah, etc.)

## Purposes

{ Provides a forum to discuss controversial topics.
{ Provides new ideas for teaching.

---

**Advantages**

- Provides audience participation.
- Can be adapted for use by someone else.
- Has both positive and negative aspects.
- Is a familiar format for TV watchers.

**Disadvantages**

- Uniquely developed by Donahue.
- May be viewed primarily as entertainment.
- Needs to be understood and modified by the teacher.
- Can be confusing if not organized well.

---

## Suggestions for Use

### Techniques from Passe (page 43)

1. Studies the issue before the show.
2. Presents an intriguing background analysis before eliciting comments.
3. Relaxes his participants.
4. Avoids embarrassing anyone.
5. Keeps the discussion moving.
6. Rewords any comments that might be misunderstood.
7. Prevents anyone from monopolizing or going off on tangents.
8. Encourages participants to speak about their feelings.
9. Uses humor to lower tension.
10. Asks good questions.

### Pointers from Huff (page 230)

1. If you're presenting a subject to a group, keep the dialogue conversational. Don't let intense feelings burst into flames. Keep the subject moving around the room.
2. Clarify carefully -- credit merit. Respect your resisters. Be a good distiller. "Isn't *this* what we're really trying to say here...?"
3. Make an honest effort to get everybody involved. Reach out to them.
4. Protect the soft-spoken and inarticulate. Don't let the big talkers clobber the people who can't get their thoughts out. Direct traffic.
5. Have a good time. But demonstrate that you're really involved in this subject -- and that the truth is going to serve, perhaps even *save*, them all.

**References**


Murray, B., & Copeland, L. (1992). Is there a place for Phil Donahue in the classroom? Journal of Nursing Education, 31, 285-286.

Passe, J. (1984). Phil Donahue: An excellent model for leading a discussion. Journal of Teacher Education, 35, 43-48.

Huff, R. (1992). "I can see you naked": A fearless guide to making great presentations(2nd ed.). Kansas City: Andrews & McMeel.

## TANKA

### Definition

*Tanka* is a Japanese fixed form of 5-line verse, of 31 syllables (5-7-5-7-7).

### Purposes

- Provide a creative, original form of poetry.
- Increase understanding and empathy of issues and topics.
- Teach a Japanese free verse poetry form.

---

**Advantages**

- Demonstrates a creative form of poetry.
- Has been in continued use since the 8th century.
- Provides a form of expression available to those who find difficulty with verbal expression.
- Simple to write.
- Poems written by others may be read.

**Disadvantages**

- Requires knowledge of basic rules.
- May be viewed by learners as less than educational.

---

### Points to Remember

- Flow of individual lines or groups of lines given more importance than mathematical tabulation of sounds.
- Originally love poems, but may express many emotions and moods.
- If teacher does not wish to assist learners to write their own, may wish to use what others have written (including those translated from Japanese).
- When teaching how to write tanka, examples may be useful, such as:

It is fortunate
for any man who can
live so long to hear
The sound of his wife's voice
till his black hair turns to white

If from your mouth
there hung a hundred-year-old tongue
and you would babble
I still would not cease to care
but indeed my love would grow

**Other Related Methodologies:** Haiku, Cinquains.

## References

Man 'Yoshu. (1979). Ten thousand leaves. Boulder, CO: Shambhala Publishers.

# TERM PAPER

## Definition

*Term Paper* is an essay or written discussion of a subject in partial fulfillment of the requirements of a course.

## Purposes

- Encourages creative work by learner.
- Provide learner with opportunity for integration and synthesis.
- Provide teacher with chance to see progress, literary skills, and evaluate student's work.

---

| | |
|---|---|
| **Advantages** | • Permits student to work independently.<br>• Allows for selection of a subject that interests the learner.<br>• Can be individualized. |
| **Disadvantages** | • May be largely theoretical, not applicable.<br>• May be an overused method of learning and evaluation.<br>• Guidelines may not be clear.<br>• Evaluation and grading may be confused and ambiguous. |

---

## Points to Remember

- Select the method because it fits with the objectives.
- Provide criteria when assignment is given initially and/or periodically.
- Provide periodic assistance as appropriate to course and learner level.
- Distinguish between evaluation and grading.

**Other Related Methodologies:** Project, Homework.

## References


Blaga, J. (1977, June/July). Say good-bye to those dumb old term papers. Audio Visual Instructor, 22(6), 16-18.

Elbe, K. (1976). The craft of teaching. San Francisco: Jossey-Bass Publications.

Petrowski, D. (1978, September). The term paper revisited. Journal of Nursing Education, 17(7), 50-52.

Tigerman, N. (1979). 50 favorite reasons for late term papers. Nursing Outlook, 27(7), 469.

# TOUR (non-guided)

## Definition

*Non-guided Tour* is a walking tour by an individual for a specific purpose and usually with specific instructions.
Synonym -- self tour, orientation tour, scavenger hunt, tour-guided walking tour.

## Purposes

- Permit individuals to learn via touring on their own initiative.
- Allow the instructor to prepare for but not participate in repetitive tours.
- Orient adults to a facility, individuals, or equipment at their own convenience.

---

## Advantages

- Allows individual to schedule time and determine pace; may repeat.
- Stimulate curiosity and interest in a new situation.
- Involves learner in activity with guidelines provided by teacher.
- Places, people, and materials are observable in their usual location.
- Reduces cost and teacher time since teacher is freed from accompanying individual and/or groups on a tour they may complete unassisted.
- Less disruptive of ongoing operations if individuals come at intervals rather than groups.
- May be combined with other media -- visual media (such as maps, charts, posters, photographs), cassette tape and slide-tape presentations.

## Disadvantages

- Requires initiative and responsibility of learners.
- Requires careful planning by teacher.
- Learners may be distracted or miss key points or locations.
- Learners may be lost, discouraged, or dislike the solo activity.

---

## Points to Remember

- Teacher needs to plan carefully based on objectives.
- Teacher should "take" the tour before the students and plan with departments or individuals who will be observed and/or potentially inconvenienced by the tour.
- Consider most useful instructions, any restrictions, and what aids will enhance the self tour.
- Prepare and place maps, charts, posters, and photographs strategically and carefully.
- Suggest amount of time required to complete the tour, and best time of day or week to accomplish if appropriate.

- Determine whether or not discussion is necessary following tour and if tour must be completed prior to any discussion date.
- Review and evaluate the tour and value of tour, including the learner's evaluation.

**Other Related Methodologies:** Field Trip, Studycade.

**References**


Gustafson, M. (1908). Be your own tour guide. Journal of Continuing Education in Nursing 41, 51-53.

Kimmel, J. (1975). Turn left at the morgue. Inservice Training and Education 4(4), 22-26. (A description of orientation techniques for new workers in a county hospital.)

# TRIVIA/TRIVIAL PURSUIT

## Definition

*Trivia* means having a hidden significance, unimportant matters, trifles, common.
*Trivial Pursuit* is a popular commercial board game, introduced in 1993.

## Purposes

- Capitalize on a popular game as creative teaching strategy
- Plan for learning to be fun, and stimulate interest in topics otherwise thought boring.
- Develop for specific topic or content.

---

**Advantages**

- Utilize a well-known format of games for teaching purposes.
- Can be prepared by either the teacher of students.
- Provides experiential experience.
- Use of gaming promotes active learning.

**Disadvantages**

- Requires preparation time, equipment and supplies.
- Can be competitive.

---

## Ready Made Games

1. Clinical Laboratory Trivia (Medical Dimensions, Inc., 451 Reflection Road, Apple Valley, MN 55124)
2. Nursing Trivia (Nursing Trivia, Box 3616-D, Milford CT 06460)

## References


Barber-Madden, R., & Glanz, K. (1989). Participatory learning in continuing nursing education: Soviet edition of a public health and medicine trivia game. Journal of Continuing Education in Nursing, 20, 128-131.

Cooper, S. (1989). Teaching tips: Creative teaching strategies. Journal of Continuing Education in Nursing, 20, 95-96.

Fitzgerald, L., & McCurren, C. (1988). In pursuit of accreditation. Nursing and Health Care, 9, 143-145.

Gustafson, M. (1991). Board game with a health focus. Health World, 2 (8), 13-14.

Hartsock, J., & Lange, R. (1981). Trivia games. Stimulating students' learning. Nursing Educator, 12, 24-27.

# VALUE CLARIFICATION STRATEGIES

**Definition**

*Value Clarification Strategies* is an approach that can be used to help another person choose, prize (feel good about and share), and take action to clarify values. The focus of this strategy is on the process of valuing, not on the content of the values.

**Purposes**

- Encourages each person to examine her own values.
- Approaches objectives in the affective domain. Incorporates search for value along with search for knowledge.
- Applies critical thinking to matters largely in the affective domain.
- Encourages consideration of alternative modes of thinking and acting.
- Weights the consequences of alternative courses of action.

---

**Advantages**

- Provides a structured way to help students explore the connection between what they perceive as their beliefs, and their own feelings, opinions, and behavior.
- Easy strategy forces listeners to make choices, then examine them.
- Questions are short and quickly evoke feelings and opinions.
- Strategies can be adapted to content areas and specific situations.
- Subjects may be chosen to focus on one process (choosing, prizing, or acting) or on the entire value process.
- Strategies have many possible uses: introduction to classes, summary of or stimulus for discussion, etc.
- Time required is flexible and variable.

**Disadvantages**

- The value clarification approach as developed by Louis Raths assumes that the teacher is not concerned with the "content" of people's values, only with the process of valuing.
- It's difficult for a teacher to be impartial and promote the valuing process without interjecting her own values.
- If particular values are intended outcomes of learning, what values are chosen? Who selects the "right" values?
- Values may unintentionally be imposed.
- Negative attitudes may be developed if strategies are not used appropriately.
- There is controversy about value clarification and its humanistic base.

---

## Points to Remember

- Choose a strategy that suits the purpose. (The book Values Clarification: A Handbook of Practical Strategies for Teachers and Students gives many strategies that can be used or modified).
- Think about which of the seven processes of valuing (as described by Raths) is required by the strategy. Example:
  Choosing
    1) Freely.
    2) From alternatives.
    3) After considering consequences.
  Prizing
    1) Feeling good about choice.
    2) Sharing the choice.
  Acting
    1) Doing something about the choice.
    2) Repeating the action.
- Be sure to allow time for thought and discussion.
- Use questions to encourage further examination of ideas and use of the valuing processes.
- Guide thinking along new lines, but not necessarily toward specific answers, unless
- particular values are desired.
- The aim is to clarify values, not instill any particular beliefs or principles.

## Examples of Strategy

Would you rather be --

Rich?
Famous?
Healthy?
Happy?

## References


Barrett, J. (1978). Values clarification as a teaching strategy in nursing. Journal of Nursing Education, 17(2), 12-18.

Coletta, S. (1978). Values clarification in nursing: Why? American Journal of Nursing, 78(12), 2057.

Corcoran, S. (1975). The value of values in nursing education. Image, 7(3), 5-9.

Cznowski, M. (1974). Value teaching in nursing. Nursing Forum, 12(2), 192-206.

Dressel, P. L. (1971). Values, cognitive and affective. Journal of Higher Education, 42, 400-405.

Hall, B. P. (1973). Value clarification as learning process: A source book. New York: Paulist Press.

Harmin, M., Kirschenbaum, H., & Simon, S. (1973). Teaching subject matter with a focus on values. Minneapolis: Winston Press.

Raths, L., Harmin, M., & Simon, S. (1966). Values and teaching: Working with values in the classroom. Columbus, OH: Charles E. Merrill Books, Inc. (Emphasizes theory and application of value clarification.)

Simon, S., Howe, L., & Kirschenbaum, H. (1972). Values clarification: A handbook of practical strategies for teachers and students. New York: Hart Publishing Co. (Gives strategies for value clarification.)

Dewey, J. (1939). Theory of valuation. Chicago: University of Chicago Press.

Gordon, T. (1970). Parent effectiveness training. New York: Peter H. Wyden.

Kirschenbaum, H., Simon, S., & Napier, R. (1971). Wad-Ja-Get? The grading game in American education. New York: Hart Publishing.

Krathwohl, D., et al. Taxonomy of educational objectives, Handbook II: Affective domain. New York: David McKay, Co.

Manning, D. (1971). Toward a humanistic curriculum. New York: Harper and Row.

Maslow, A. (1959). New knowledge in human values. New York: Harper and Row.

Metcalf, L. (1971). Values education. Washington, D.C.: National Council for Social Studies.

Uustal, D. (1978). Values clarification in nursing: Application to practice. AMerican JOURNAL of NURSING, 78(12), 2058-2-63.

# VIDEOS

## Definition

*Videos* are a reproduction of television pictures on standard magnetic tape. The material recorded on such tape is played back in audiovisual form on a television receiver with video cassette player (VCR).

## Purposes

- Individual or group learning.
- Documentation of events or activities.
- Self evaluation for achievement of objectives.
- More objective evaluation of performance, can replay to validate data.
- Demonstration of particular skill or approaches.

---

**Advantages**

- Replay possible, allows viewing of self in actual situation.
- Can be viewed in formal setting or at home.
- Tapes are erasable and reusable.
- Can compare "early" and "later" performance to determine progress.
- Can observe effects of own behavior on others.

**Disadvantages**

- Cost of equipment and tapes, initial purchase, maintenance and storage.
- Need technician or someone who is familiar with equipment and able to run it.
- May be threatening to participants.
- Time consuming to develop.
- Professional looking videos may be costly to develop.

---

## Teacher's Responsibilities

- Determine appropriateness of method for objectives.
- Clarify purpose of video use to learners.
- Able to use method effectively (operate equipment, if no technician available).
- If using video taping to evaluate student's performance...
  a. prepare students -- may be hesitant to see themselves of video.
  b. may want to video tape class session or teacher before doing it with individual students.
  c. specify level of expectation.
  d. ask permission of students to be taped -- don't force.
  e. might have student participate in planning for use.
  f. be explicit about how, why, and for whom it will be used (only for students' viewing, or others).

g. might briefly explain equipment. If other people are involved in the video tapes, i.e., patients, be sure to prepare them as well and obtain written permission for the taping.

**References**


Berger, M. M. (Ed.). (1970). Video tape techniques in psychiatric training and treatment. New York: Brunner, Mazel Publications.

Good, C. V. (1973). Dictionary of education (3rd ed.). New York: McGraw-Hill).

Koch, H. (1975). Film or television? Nursing Outlook, 23(1). (A comparison of films and TV in terms of production and use.)

Koch, H. (1968). Television in nursing education. Journal of Nursing Education, 7(2), 37-43.

Lorena, C. (1973). To tape ourselves as others see us. Inservice Training and Education, 1(2), 26-30.

Mrucke, M. (1970). Videotape recordings: A tool for psychiatric clinical supervision. Perspectives in Psychiatric Care, 8(5), 200-208.

Shaffer, M. K., & Pfeiffer, I. (1976). Television can improve instruction. Journal of Nursing Education, 15(6), 3-8.

Shaffer, M., & Pfeiffer, I. (1980). You too can prepare videotapes for instruction. Journal of Nursing Education, 19(3), 23-27.

Simonda, A. (1970). Two methods of teaching in the O.R. Nursing Outlook, 18(2). (Videotape playback and audio tutorial methods are compared.)

Some video do's and don'ts for the do-it-yourselfer. (1973). Inservice Training and Education, 1(2), 42. (A helpful list of pointers covering purchasing, maintaining and preparing for taping, camera work, editing and handling and storage of tapes.)

10 a.m. Channel 6: Cardiac nursing with our own Miss Smith. (1973). Inservice Training and Education, 1(2), 32. (Videotaping is being discussed by a hospital education and training programmer.)

# WORKSHOP

## Definition

*Workshop* is a type of meeting that offers opportunities for persons with a common interest or problem to meet with specialists to receive firsthand knowledge and practice. A series of individual sessions.

## Purposes

- Provide a group of individuals the opportunity to explore an area of interest through a series of sessions or presentations.
- Give individuals opportunity to receive help from other participants and resource people.
- Provide learning situations based on the interests and needs of participants.
- Provide group learning situations in general sessions and subgroup meetings of various sizes for various purposes.

---

## Advantages

- All workshops are participate.
- Participants identify their interests and needs and the learning situations are based on these.
- Large numbers can be accommodated.
- Allows for flexibility
- Emphasis is on improving the individual's understanding and proficiency.
- "Theory" and "practice" may be considered concurrently.
- Individuals are encouraged to work out their own tasks, and assistance is available.

## Disadvantages

- Individuals may not perceive that their needs were identified initially, or met during the course of the sessions.
- In order to maximize use of time, much needs to be considered in planning and organizing.
- Some learners may find it more difficult to learn with this format.
- It may be an overused methodology for some groups or participants.
- Selection of resource people may be difficult.
- Last minute changes affect a large number of learners.
- The session may not "flow" well or be interrelated.

---

**Individuals Involved in a Workshop:**

Participants -- those for whom the workshop is planned. May or may not be required to pay a fee or prepare in advance.

Coordinator (or director) -- offers leadership or guidance throughout, as well as planning of the sessions. May or may not be responsible for:

a. Setting up committees.
b. Orientation of resource persons and leaders.
c. Liaison with sponsors (and publicity).

Resource persons -- present information and authoritative opinion in general sessions and/or in subgroups.

a. Make systematic presentations (speech, symposium, demonstration).
b. May lead discussions groups or sessions.
c. In practice groups, may show how to carry out procedure and offer opportunity for participants to practice procedure.

Staff -- may act alternately as instructors, discussion leaders, and/or resource persons (This may refer to secretarial staff and include tasks like transcriber, registration, moderator, etc.).

**Responsibilities of Coordinator or Director**

- Arrange topic after assessment of needs and interests of those who will attend.
- Design the workshop:

  Establish objectives.

  1) Participants must be able to "learn" or "do" something.
  2) Relate "something" closely to that which occurs on the job and is practical.
  3) Consider learnings that should occur pre-, during-, and post-workshop.
  4) Determine if practice sessions are necessary during the workshop.

  Develop the basic plan.

  1) Determine:
     a) what will be presented.
     b) what will be discussed.
     c) what will be practiced.
  2) Consider subgroup activities and size.
     a) small interest groups, 15-20.
     b) work groups, 10-25.
     c) discussion groups, 10-20.
     d) practice groups, 10-15.
  3) Consider materials which need to be prepared for the participants.
     a) handbook.
     b) discussion guides.
     c) practice instructions and/or diagrams.
     d) quizzes.

4) Determine equipment needed.
   a) chalkboards
   b) overhead visuals
   c) demonstration devices
   d) videos
5) determine room arrangements.

Select the best method.
1) Consider the selected techniques with the schedule and budget.
2) Determine "who" should do what.

Expand outline.
1) Meet with resource people as needed, provide them with materials.
2) Review with committee those tasks delegated.

Plan for evaluation.
1) Plan for evaluation (by the participants) of each presenter and for each selected session and/or activities.
2) Plan for a verbal and/or written review session by resource persons and leaders (may include committee members).
3) Keep a file of evaluations and sample materials for future reference and/or duplication of workshop.

**Other Related Methodologies:** Seminar, Institute, Conference.

**References**


Bergevin, P., et al. (1963). Adult education procedures (pp. 223-225). New York: Seabury Press. (A brief section, very readable.)

Davis, L., & McCallon, E. (1974). Planning, conducting and evaluating workshops. Austin, TX: Learning Concepts.

Elliott, H. L. (1970). A traction workshop for orderlies. Nursing Outlook, 18(3), 47. (One example from nursing.)

Friedman, W., et al. (1979). Work shopping. Nurse Educator, 4(6), 19-22.

Gerber, R. (1980). The mini-workshop. Nursing Outlook, 28(2), 126-127.

Parker, B., Pierce, M., & Sturm, I. E. (1975). Evaluating a workshop method for teaching the problem-oriented record to nurses. Journal of Continuing Education in Nursing 6(3), 34-39. (The teaching group of a one-day workshop at a VA hospital in New York report their approach and findings.)

Rebedeau, F. C. (1975). Developing a sales training workshop session. Training and Development Journal, 29(11), 12-16. (A helpful "how to" article from a major corporation.)

Smith, C. (1977). Identifying blocks to communication in health care settings and a workshop. Journal of Continuing Education in Nursing 8(2), 26-32.

Smyth, Sister K., & McMahon, J. (1976). A workshop approach to continuing education. Nurse Educator, 1(4), 16-20. (The description of "how to" collaboratively plan a continuing education program for nurses.)

Stevens, B. J. (1977). The successful workshop: How to bring it off!! Nurse Educator, 2(1), 16-20. (Some practical suggestions for both sponsors and leaders of workshops, interestingly written.)

Wolf, M., & Coggins, C. (1987). A workshop for development of simulation games in nursing. Journal of Continuing Education in Nursing 12(3), 31-34.